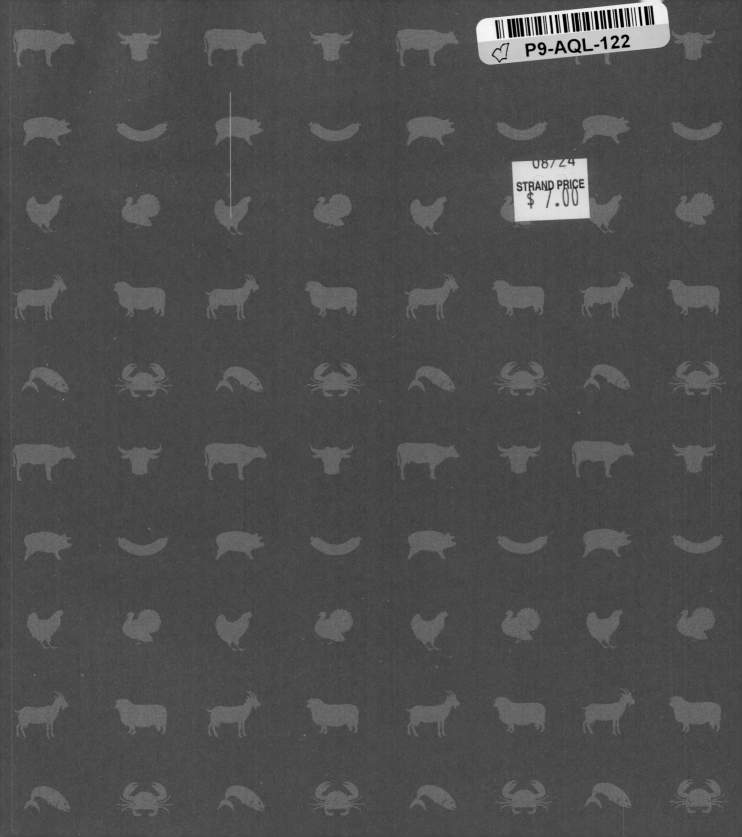

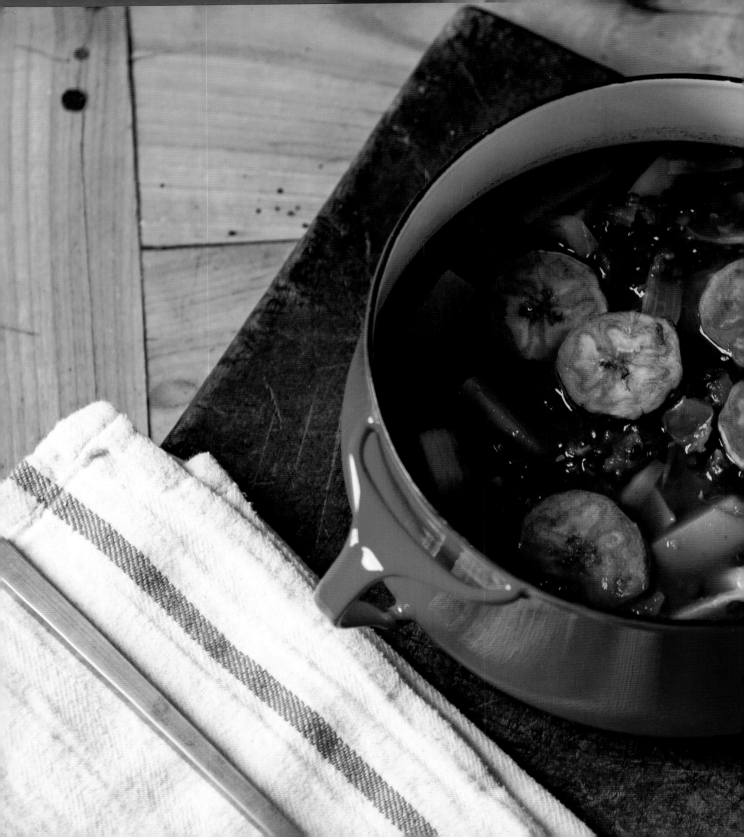

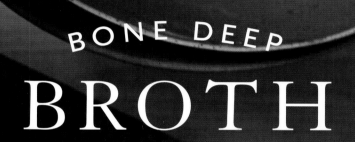

BONE DEEP
BROTH

HEALING RECIPES
with BONE BROTH

Taylor Chen & Lya Mojica

OWNERS OF BONE DEEP & HARMONY

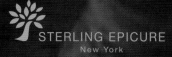

STERLING EPICURE
New York

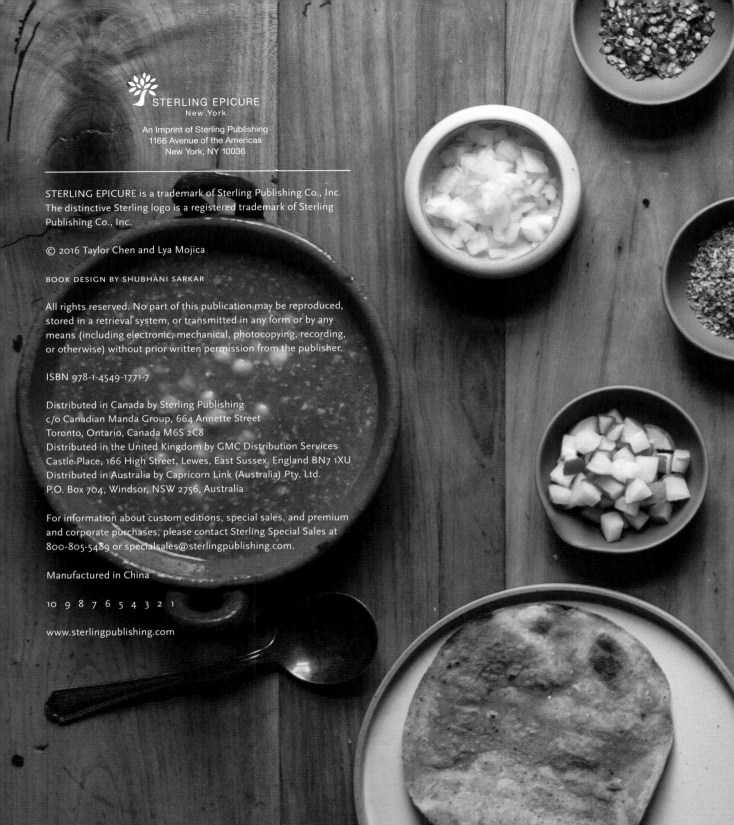

STERLING EPICURE
New York

An Imprint of Sterling Publishing
1166 Avenue of the Americas
New York, NY 10036

BOOK DESIGN BY SHUBHANI SARKAR

ISBN 978-1-4549-1771-7

Distributed in Canada by Sterling Publishing
c/o Canadian Manda Group, 664 Annette Street
Toronto, Ontario, Canada M6S 2C8
Distributed in the United Kingdom by GMC Distribution Services
Castle Place, 166 High Street, Lewes, East Sussex, England BN7 1XU
Distributed in Australia by Capricorn Link (Australia) Pty. Ltd.
P.O. Box 704, Windsor, NSW 2756, Australia

For information about custom editions, special sales, and premium
and corporate purchases, please contact Sterling Special Sales at
800-805-5489 or specialsales@sterlingpublishing.com.

Manufactured in China

10 9 8 7 6 5 4 3 2 1

www.sterlingpublishing.com

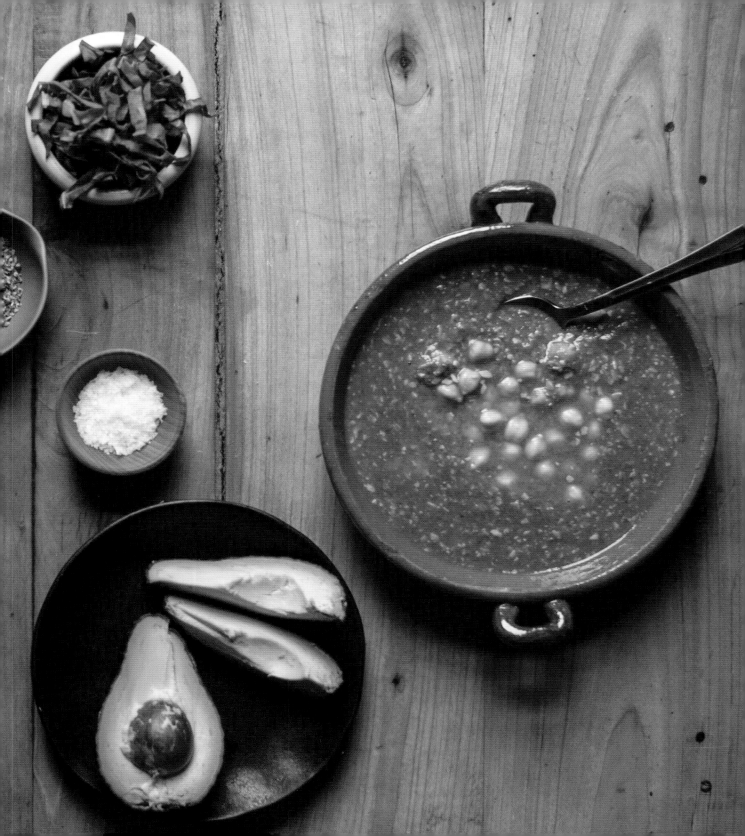

CONTENTS

Bone Broth: The Basics

Recipes

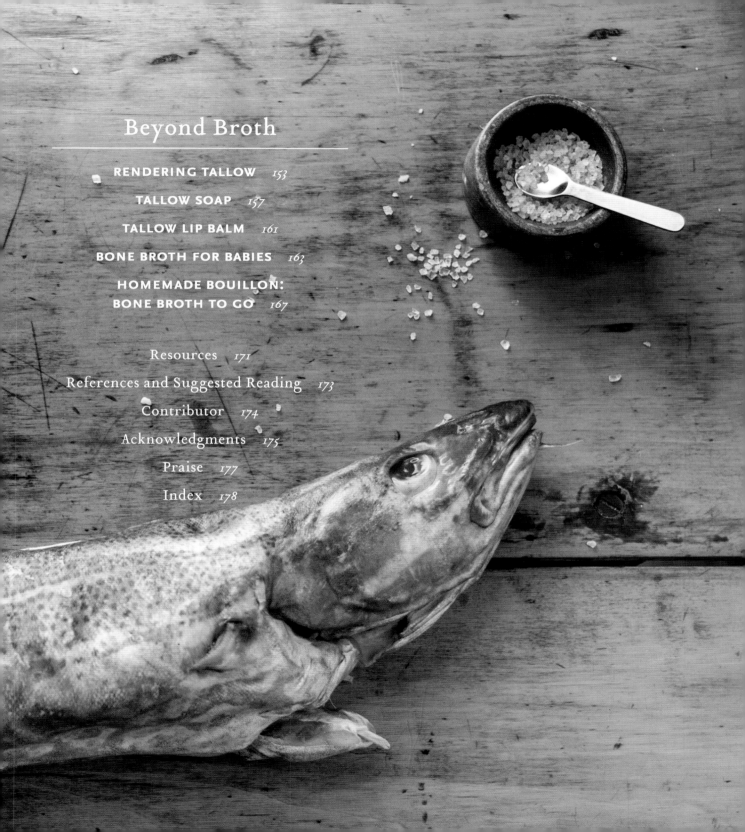

Beyond Broth

Foreword

WHAT'S OLD IS NEW, THAT'S HOW THE SAYING GOES.

Lya and Taylor take a timeless food, bone broth, and deliver it to a new generation with simple, straightforward, and easy to digest information and recipes. It's an educational and culinary treasure. Food is more than sustenance; it is legacy, heritage, and possesses great healing power. Lya and Taylor's personal stories about bone broth reflect that, and it is a privilege to witness their journey and enjoy their recipes.

I grew up, as I think many people of my generation and older did, with someone always at home. Whether it was a mother or a grandmother or extended family, I learned how to cook and plan meals from them. Someone shopped every day or every other day, especially for the dinner meal. Because of that, I learned about the value of wholesome food. My parents were of first generation European descent, and so much intergenerational wisdom, or old wives' tales, was passed on through food-lore as I called it.

Through the decades of nutritional science, we have come to find out the benefit of what older generations inherently knew. Since many in recent generations have not experienced learning about food-lore through their own upbringing, everyone should be grateful to have Lya and Taylor bring them this information.

Whether I was watching my grandmother make chicken stock and breaking the softened bones to release the marrow or familiarizing myself with the benefits of primitive diets written about by Weston A.

Price, DDS, the power of nutrition was never lost on me.

As the last several decades brought everyone out of their kitchens and away from the wonders of food and toward a reliance on processed foodstuffs, chronic disease has flourished, leading many back to healing foods such as bone broth. Societally, we have burdened our bodies so much that we reached a tipping point; it's not at all sustainable or maintainable economically from a healthcare or education standpoint.

Enlightenment is occurring and people are returning to their kitchens. The cure is in the cupboard is another old adage that comes to mind, in this case, it is in the pot. As much recent science has determined, when the gut is healed, you can help heal the whole body because the gut is really the seat of the immune system and neurological system, which of course now gets a lot more press in terms of the gut-brain connection.

At the cornerstone of many popular healing diets comes the need for bone broths. So that rolls the clock back to those stocks and those broths that were an inherent part of my growing up. They take time to prepare and cook, with love and gratitude, and represent the quintessential slow food vs. fast food. I am pleased it's gotten popular as a stand-alone, with many appreciating its virtues and benefits. Taylor and Lya are truly amazing carriers of the torch.

The nutritional benefits of bone broth apropos to its

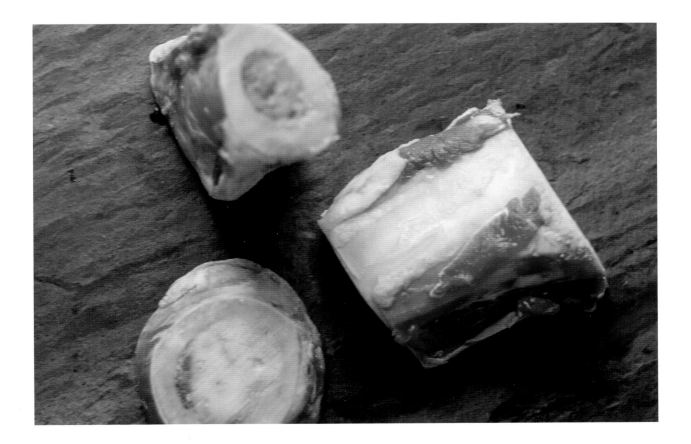

nutrient density cannot be overstated. Nutrients, like the amino acid glutamine, foundational to rebuilding a gastrointestinal tract compromised when the body is under stress, and necessary to support the production of detoxifying antioxidants, are just one example of bone broth's healing factors. The amino acid glycine is present too, and glutamine and glycine are two of the amino acids that the body uses to make glutathione, which is its primary detoxifying antioxidant. So it's really significant to help us from a detox standpoint, as well as nourishing.

Another amino acid, one folks may be more familiar with as a component of colostrum, is proline, which also makes an appearance in bone broth.

Whether one is growing, repairing or trying to stave off the aging process, collagen and minerals foundational in the broth makes this elixir a necessary component of the human diet, with all due respect to our vegan population. These are just a few examples and Lya and Taylor will delight you with informative wisdom in the following pages.

With honor and privilege, I commend Lya and Taylor on a job well done. Here is to health and wellness. Lift your cup of bone broth!

Geri Brewster, RDN MPH
CLINICAL NUTRITIONIST
FOUNDER OF BUILDYOURBESTBUMP.COM

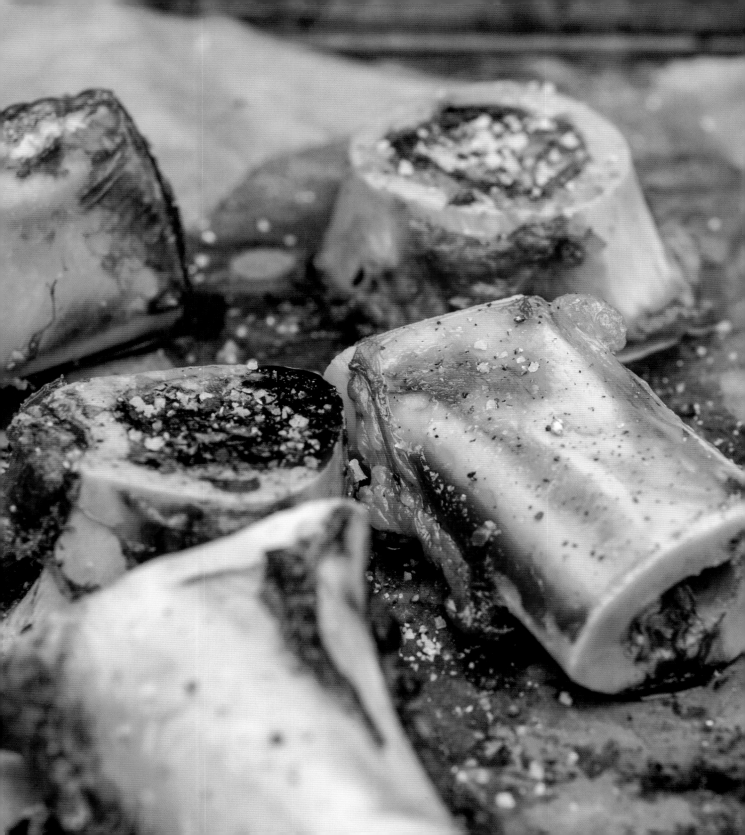

Overview and Introduction to Bone Broth

BONE BROTH IS BY NO MEANS A RECENT TREND. It is an ancient superfood that is simple, delicious, and effective. It has been a mainstay among traditional cultures worldwide for thousands of years as a healing aid. If you have ever used chicken soup to help get over a cold, you have already participated in an ancient lineage of food wisdom! Bone broth is a true tonic when properly produced. It starts with the bones of locally sourced grass-fed cows, sheep, or pasture-raised pigs and poultry, or the bones and heads of wild-caught fish. The broth is slow simmered for many hours to maximize the extraction of beneficial amino acids and minerals. Bones are the deepest and densest tissue of the body. To cook with bones is to cook with the "roots"—the core of the animals. Broth has a soothing and fortifying effect in the body, strengthening us from the core to the surface.

A well-prepared bone broth is a delightful experience for the senses. Bone broth's umami taste—the savory flavor that makes food taste delicious—is derived from the glutamates that are released during the simmering process. A study by Agostini et al has shown that the glutamates in bone broth naturally occur in similar concentrations to those in breast milk. It is no wonder that bone broth is a comfort food for humans.

Broth is the base of many traditional recipes. Imagine French cuisine and all its sauces without broths or stocks. Many Asian and African cultures begin their day using broth as the base to make porridges and soups for breakfast. Borscht in Russia is prepared with beef broth, matzo ball soup in Jewish culture is prepared with chicken broth, miso soup in Japan is prepared with fish broth, and the traditional Mexican hominy soup pozole is simmered in pork broth. What would delicious ramen soups taste like without the pork bones that flavor their broth?

The use of bones in the kitchen is a practice that is true to the principles of a holistic approach to life. From an economical and energetic point of view, it is a sustainable practice because it makes use of the part of the animals we eat that so often goes to waste. The price of bones is lower than that of muscle and organ meats. While time consuming, the process of making broth involves only a few elements: water, bones, sometimes an acid medium that will help extract most nutrients from the bones, and fire. Additional aromatics— produce, herbs, and spices—boost flavor and enhance the broth's healing capacity, for example, the addition of fennel seeds to promote lactation for nursing mothers.

From a health perspective, bone broth is a tried and true food that helps heal many conditions because it helps restore the lining of the gut. The latest research in medicine and psychology points to a disrupted GI tract, or what is called leaky gut, as the root of many modern ailments and diseases. Western medicine now affirms that most autoimmune conditions come as a result of inflammatory conditions caused by proteins that have sneaked into the bloodstream because of a leaky gut. Autoimmune conditions (allergies, thyroid and skin imbalances, infertility, and a myriad of common digestive disorders, such as IBS, colitis, and gastritis, have all been effectively treated with programs that include bone broth. Collagen in bones, concentrated in the cartilage and connective tissues, is transformed into gelatin during the simmering process of making broth. The gelatin in the broth, in turn, becomes a healing aid in restoring the health of the gastrointestinal lining.

Consequently, as the lining of the gut is restored, symptoms are reduced and the condition improves.

From a culinary perspective, bone broth imparts incomparable depth of flavor and texture to meals. It can be the starting point to a meal: a cup of broth as the first course, like a consommé, to prepare the palate and the digestive system to receive more complex foods. It is also used as a building block to prepare soups, stews, and sauces.

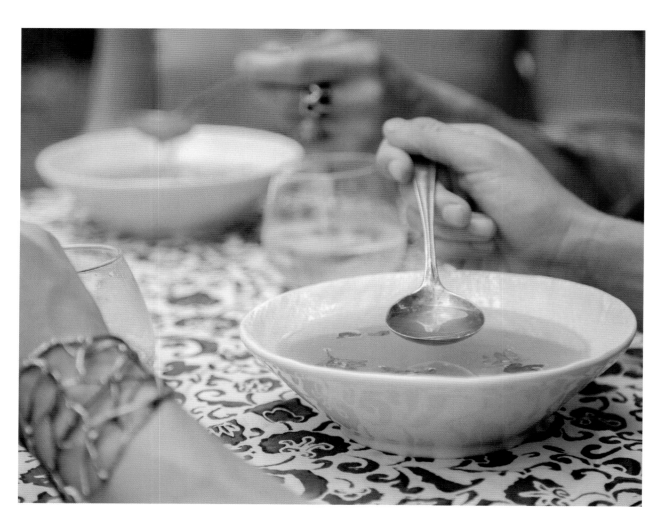

Bone Deep & Harmony

WHILE WE BOTH HAD DIFFERENT JOURNEYS ON our way to loving bone broth, it was similar experiences that connected us and led to the creation of Bone Deep & Harmony. Through the years, our spiritual- and health-focused paths led us to experiment with many trendy and plant-based diets. What we noticed was, most often, these diets focused on elimination of ingredients. Despite our best efforts to conform, we were left feeling depleted, not only physically but mentally and emotionally as well—a far cry from the vibrant and glowing claims many diets promised. As we continued to eliminate, we found ourselves pouring money into copious supplements to compensate for all of the eliminated foods. Yet we still struggled to find energy and experienced increasing levels of anxiety. Something needed to change.

On a friend's recommendation, we were introduced to acupuncturist Chris Chen. To complement the acupuncture treatments, Chris encouraged both of us to consider some serious dietary shifts. Under his guidance, we began to change our diets, including more traditional foods and incorporating bone broth into our respective routines.

As we began to work with bones, carefully simmering, skimming, and tasting broth, we started to understand the importance of these ingredients. With Mexican and Southern roots, both rich with culinary culture, our "new" practice of making bone broth in our New York City kitchens brought back endless memories of the women in our lives who prepared fresh, healthy meals that nourished our families for generations. Along with our daily dose of broth, we quickly noticed improvements in our health. Seasonal allergies were relieved, it helped regulate hormonal changes, supported our years as nursing mothers, and helped relieve chronic anxiety.

It was only natural that we would come together and create something we both loved and benefited from. When we first started making and selling bone broth, most of our customers were patients of traditional Chinese medicine doctors and acupuncturists in New York City. Our first clients had been prescribed regular consumption of bone broth as part of their healing program, a common Chinese medicinal practice. The Chinese five element system encompasses an integral vision of the universe, with the premise that there are laws that regulate all phenomena, and that the laws of nature are also the laws of humanity, and since nature and humanity must coexist, harmony is the key to life. The five elements— wood, fire, earth, metal, and water—represent the five phases of the creative cycle: beginning, growth/ expansion, collection/introspection, reversion, and harmonizing, the latter being the phase that activates the whole cycle and repeats it.

Earth is the harmonizing element, and also the element that sets the surface or ground for all the other elements. To have one's feet firmly planted on the earth

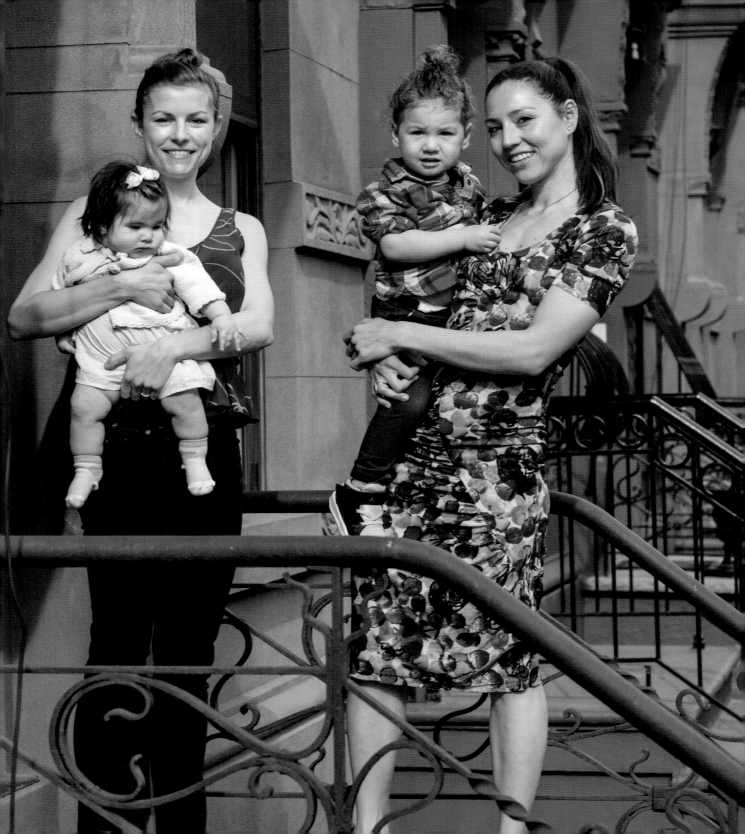

lays the foundation for a harmonious existence. The notion of the earth element as it relates to the human body became a helpful tool in our quests for balance. The Chinese system connects the earth element in our bodies with our stomach. A nourished person with a healthy digestive system has more vitality and strength to support all organ systems in the body. Chinese doctors often treat patients' earth element (that is, digestive systems) first, and bone broth is the cornerstone of developing digestive health. Like a domino effect, gradually all other systems readjust, with energy flowing throughout one's whole being.

People unfamiliar with traditional Chinese medicine were often confused when they asked what we did and we said, "We sell bone broth." They would say, "Bone . . . what? What is that?" The truth is that practically everyone knows bone broth and has most likely tasted it before. Making broth from the bones of the animals we commonly eat has been a common practice for millennia. If you are familiar with stock, you already have an idea of what bone broth is. "Really? Just bones and water? Why?" We don't blame anyone for having this reaction. We reacted the same way when we were first told that we would benefit from regular consumption of bone broth, but after incorporating it into our diets and seeing firsthand how Chris's patients were healing, we were hooked!

Having gone through the experience of using bone broth to improve our own health, we both realized that the process of making broth regularly is a challenge for many in New York City, where kitchens are pint-sized and people spend little time at home. We saw a gap in the market and decided to make broth to sell to Chris's patients. In the winter of 2013, we approached our neighborhood butcher. They were a perfect fit because they only carry locally sourced bones and meat from grass-fed cows and sheep, and pastured pork and poultry. They were responsive to

our idea and immediately began production using the recipe that we had used for years. Little did anyone know that bone broth would become the next trend in the food industry. Just months after we had been officially in business as Bone Deep & Harmony™, the bone broth hype exploded. Our commitment to the integrity of sourcing bones from small local farms that follow sustainable practices, as well as to following the old techniques of slow simmering broth, with the addition of high quality and organic ingredients, has paid off. We continue to make bone broth at home, using it as a tonic to support our well-being throughout different phases of life, especially now as parents to Elsie and Pablo.

Our hope with this cookbook is to present a fresh way of using ancient wisdom and adapting it to our times. Most of our recipes are for simple everyday meals, with the exception of a few more complex dishes that would be great for special occasions and holidays: Mole (p. 126), Yellow Thai Curry (p. 135), and Swiss Chard Rolls Filled with Braised Oxtails and Red Wine Sauce (p. 74). Broth making is time-consuming—there is no way around that. However, little active labor is involved, and if you use our basic broth preparation guidelines, you will see how easy it is. The idea is that you make large batches at a time, and if you make it a habit, it is a true joy to revel in knowing that there is broth waiting for you in the refrigerator or freezer, readily available to make a quick and nutritious homemade meal. We hope you learn to love broth as much as we do!

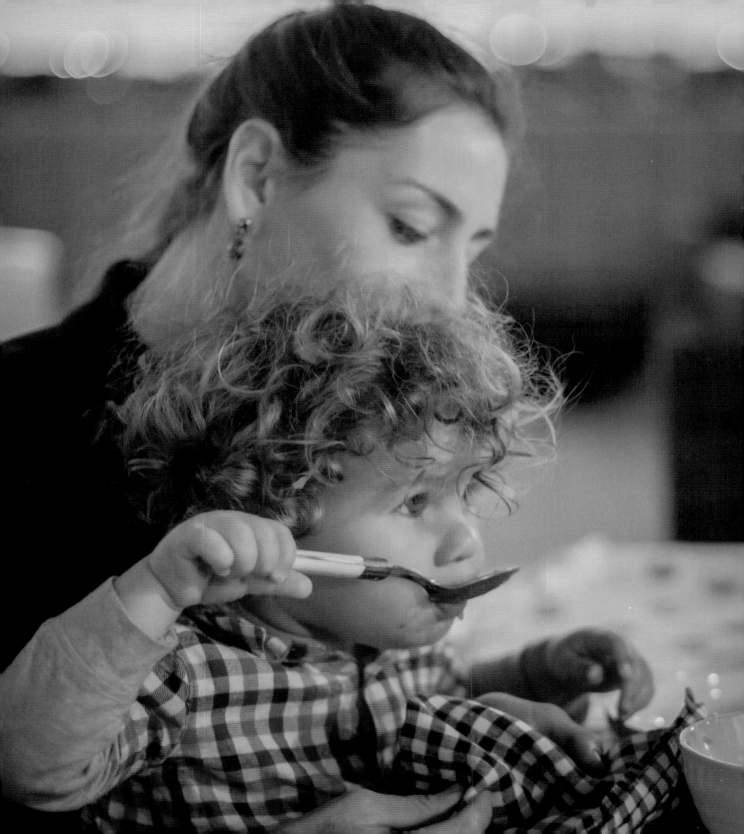

The Benefits of Bone Broth

BONE BROTH IS A TERRIFIC NOURISHING FOOD because it helps our digestive system absorb nutrients without expending too much energy. Even though broth is not high in calories, it provides many of the building blocks that our body needs to build and maintain its own structures.

The long, slow simmering of bone broth preparation allows for the optimal extraction of nutrients from the bones. We commonly add an acid, usually apple cider vinegar, to further maximize extraction. Just like our stomachs produce their own acids to break down proteins, the vinegar added in broth preparation helps break down the proteins from the bones and extract the most trace minerals.

Bone broth is a great source of many essential nutrients that our body does not manufacture on its own or that may be depleted during times of stress or illness. The nutrients in bone broth are extracted from the soft part of the bone—the marrow—as well as from the outer bone matrix, the dense part of the bone.

Bone marrow provides the most iron—the trace mineral that is at the core of hemoglobin. The iron from bone marrow is of the easily absorbable type: heme iron. Iron is essential for our bodies to transport oxygen and produce red blood cells. The bone matrix provides other trace minerals, including calcium, magnesium, phosphorus, boron, and iodine (in fish broths only). These minerals are important for healthy bones and muscles, proper nerve transmission, and gland function.

The collagen and gelatin in bone broth are of special importance in the nutrient profile and the unique therapeutic properties of bone broth. Collagen, mostly found in the cartilage and connective tissue attached to bones, though also part of the bone matrix, is reduced to gelatin during the cooking process. It helps in the formation and repair of cartilage and bone healing, and in the coating of the mucous membranes of the gastrointestinal tract. It also facilitates the digestion and assimilation of proteins, and is beneficial in reducing bruising, healing wounds quickly, and promoting healthy skin.

The amino acids found in higher concentration in bone broth are proline, glycine, glutamine, and alanine. Although these amino acids are not considered essential because our bodies can produce them, the reality is that only people who are in excellent health manufacture enough of these amino acids to satisfy their needs. Most of us need to supplement with nutrient-dense foods.

Proline and glycine are key in our own manufacture of cartilage and collagen, which give us healthy joints and skin. Glycine is key in the production of other amino acids, and it is involved in many important functions in our body: It builds our blood, it is involved in the production of glucose, it enhances gastric acid secretion, it assists in wound healing, and it plays an essential role in the detoxification process of the liver. The amino acid alanine is involved in the production of glucose and in helping with our liver's functions. It also helps with building muscle mass and is praised by athletes because it enhances physical endurance.

Glutamine is one of the most abundant amino acids in our bodies, found in the gastrointestinal tract. While our body can make glutamine itself from glutamic acid through the glutamate ammonium ligase, glutamine levels are often compromised after surgery, when under stress, and when immune function is low. This is troublesome because glutamine plays an important role in many metabolic processes: maintaining acid–alkaline balance in our systems; ensuring firm, healthy skin; promoting wound healing; assisting the detoxification process of the liver; combating fat storage from sugars; aiding our brain's production of GABA, the naturally occurring neurotransmitter commonly taken as a supplement for its calming effect on the nervous system; and enhancing our immune system. Interestingly, the gastrointestinal mucosal lining is made up of cells that feed on glutamine more than any other amino acid. Glutamine is an essential aid for gut cells to grow and heal.

GLUTAMINE, GLUTAMIC ACID, AND GLUTAMATES IN BONE BROTH

The long cooking time in the preparation of bone broth causes proteins from the bones to become unbound and to break down. One of the amino acids that becomes unbound from the proteins is glutamic acid. Glutamic acid is a nonessential amino acid (meaning that our body can synthesize it) that acts as an important neurotransmitter. A form of glutamic acid is called glutamate, and most of the glutamic acid in the body is found in the form of glutamates. Glutamates can form bonds with sodium salts, forming MSG (monosodium glutamate). MSG is naturally occurring in many foods, and it enhances the savory/meaty flavor that is known as umami. Many people are highly sensitive and negatively reactive to MSG. Symptoms range from headaches and sweating to asthma-like reactions, rapid heart palpitations, nausea, numbness, and facial tightness.

MSG is naturally occurring in bone broth, and the levels of MSG will depend on how long the broth is cooked, the temperature at which it is cooked, and the addition of vinegar. Lower temperatures, shorter cooking times, and the absence of vinegar will significantly decrease the glutamate content in the broth. On the other hand, when the broth simmers for a longer period of time (at least 24 hours) at a low temperature, and with the addition of apple cider vinegar, the more nutrients will be extracted from the bones. For those who are sensitive to MSG or who have a compromised digestive system, we suggest eliminating the vinegar in broth preparation, shortening the cooking time to 4 hours, and making sure the broth simmers at a low temperature.

Why Beef Broth Is the Foundation of Our Broth Making and Business

WE LOOK AT BROTH FROM BOTH WESTERN AND traditional Chinese medicine (TCM) perspectives, and we are fortunate to work alongside acupuncturist Chris Chen. The TCM perspective is fascinating because it includes a system of functional relationships that integrate the whole human being.

Oriental medicine has a unique way of recognizing how food enters our systems and how it is directed. When we eat a particular food, the food is distributed by the meridians and directed toward particular organs. The different foods that we eat have different channels of entry and primarily affect a set of organs.

From this perspective, cows are related to the earth element and the organs of the stomach and spleen. Cows have four stomachs, without which they would not be able to break down the grasses they eat for nourishment and energy. Because cows have extremely evolved stomach function, making broth from beef bones is a way to harness that specific energy and prepare it so the human body can benefit from the cow's naturally strong digestive energy.

Additionally, one of the measures of vitality in human beings is the general strength of their bone structure. When measuring the health of a human, we look not only at the size but density of the bones. The denser the bones, the more vital that person is—*vitality* being defined as the ability to maintain homeostasis. The most dense human has bones that don't even come close to those of the least dense cow.

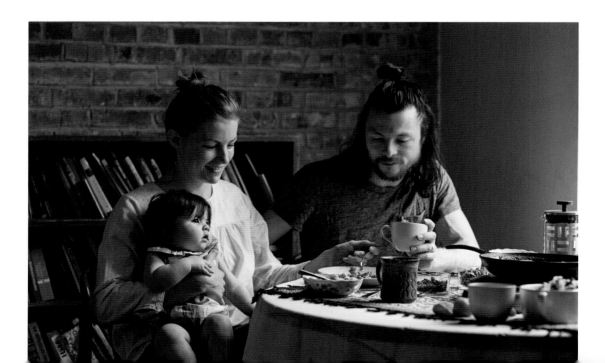

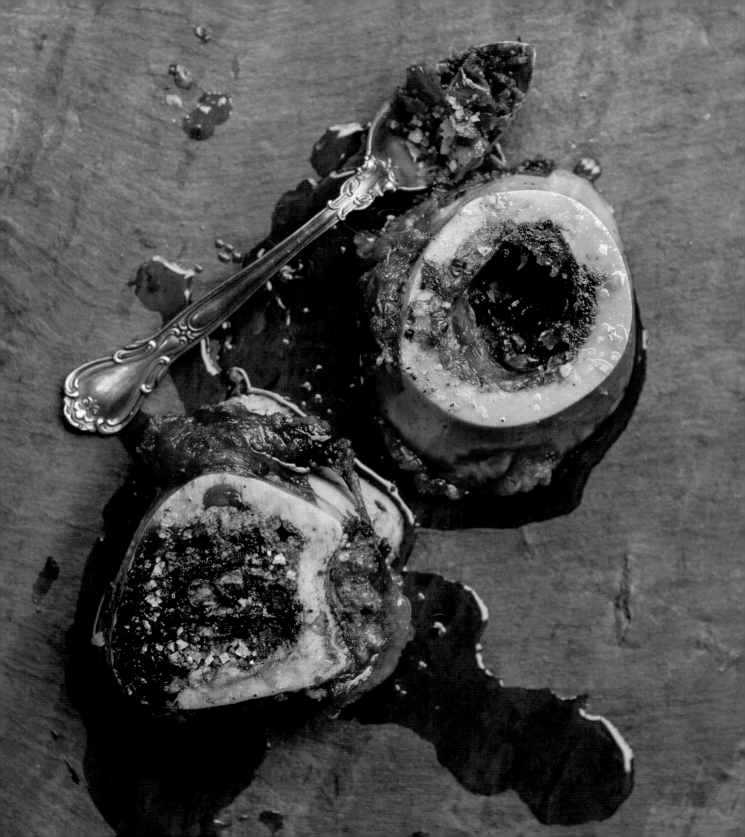

The Difference Between
Broth, Stock, and Bone Broth

WE ARE OFTEN ASKED WHAT THE DIFFERENCE IS between broth, stock, and bone broth, and there is no exact answer. Different books, blogs, and articles have different views on the meaning of each. Culinary experts tend to say that stock is made with bones and water only and minimally seasoned for use in the preparation of soups, stews, and sauces. They state that stocks are gelatinous and impart a fuller mouthfeel because of the cartilage and connective tissues attached to the bones, making stock perfect for adding texture and richness to dishes. They call broths, on the other hand, preparations of water, meat, vegetables, aromatics, and seasonings. These broths are flavorful and may be consumed on their own. They are usually clear and not necessarily gelatinous.

Others claim that stock and broth can be made using both meat and bones, but the difference is that stock is kept unseasoned and broth is seasoned. Most people use both terms interchangeably. The bone broth that has gained attention in health-minded circles, and the one we make, is a combination of all of these. We use meaty bones for flavor and nutrition. Our goal is to produce broths that are rich in gelatin for its health benefits. We add vinegar for optimal extraction of nutrients from the bones, and we use seasonings and aromatics to make the broth delicious and easy to drink on its own.

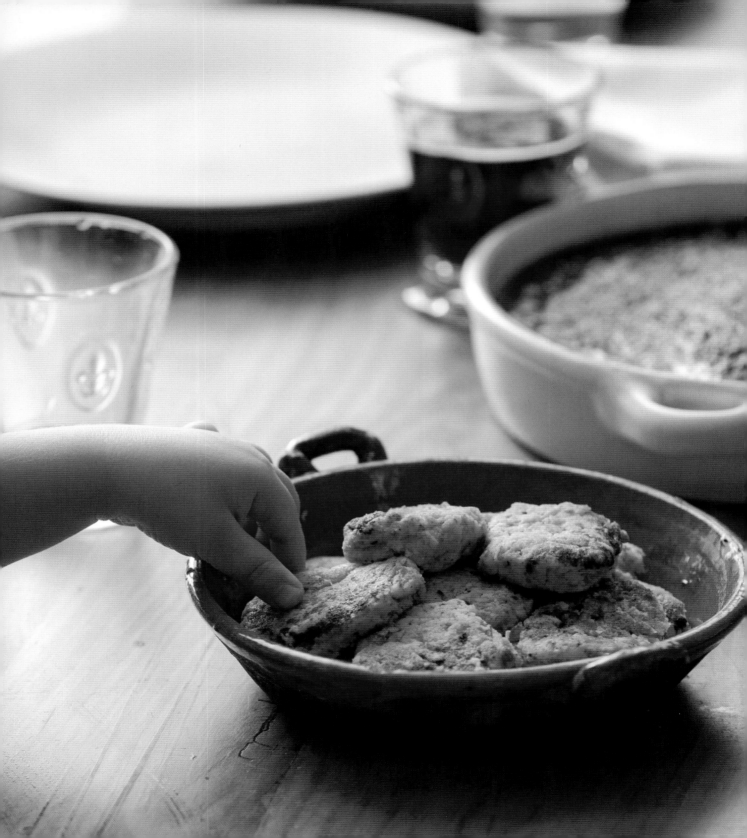

"I have been making bone broth myself for about two years. I LOVE it! I was so excited when I discovered Bone Deep & Harmony because I don't always have time to make my own, and I go through a lot of it! I have found it to be incredibly helpful for joint aches and stiffness and of course for helping to seal and repair inflammation in the gut. I also notice an overall sense of vigor and energy from eating organ meats. My favorites are beef heart and chicken liver. I eat one or the other, or sometimes both, daily."

—*Anna Venizelos,*
PROFESSIONAL ACROBAT AND CONTORTIONIST

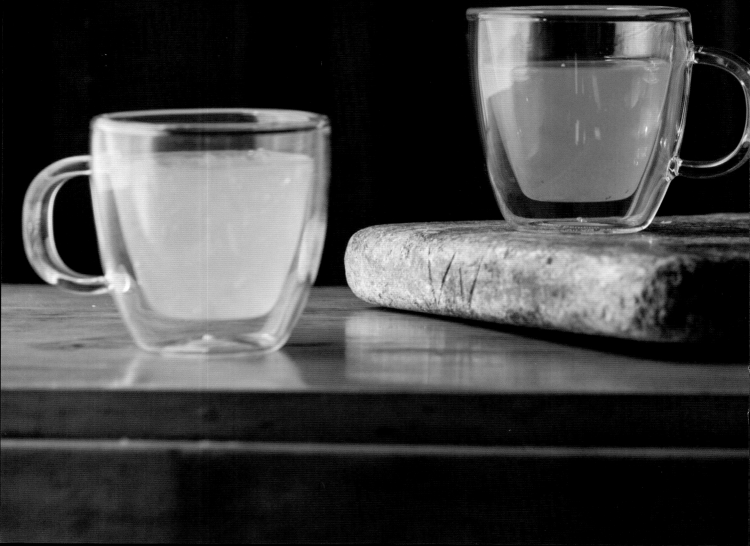

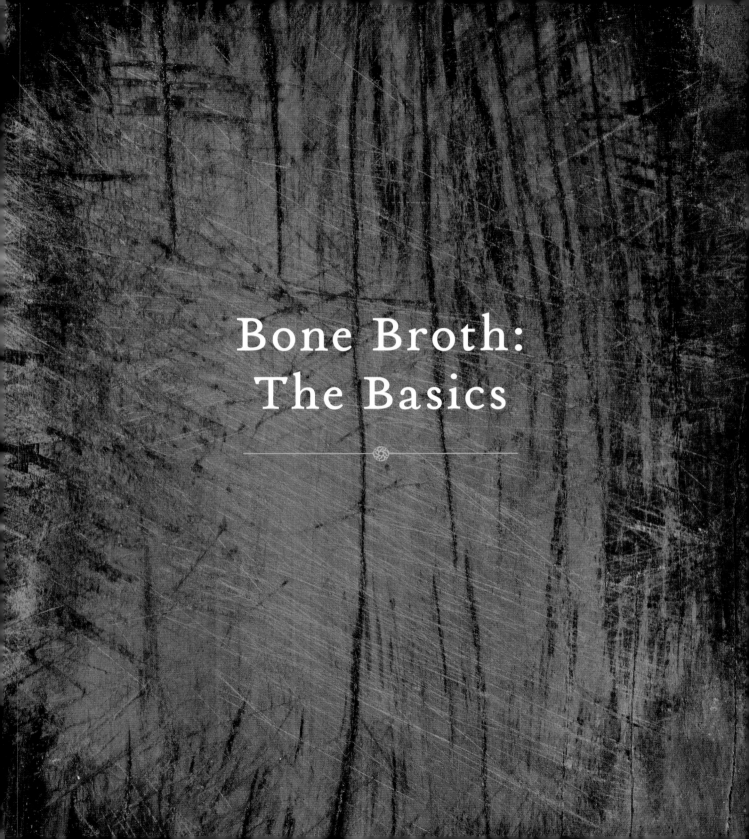

Bone Broth:
The Basics

BONE BROTH IS EASY TO MAKE, BUT IT takes a little planning and requires a long cooking time. It can, however, be made in large batches, left to cook overnight, and stored frozen for extended use. Any animal bones can be used, from chicken, turkey, duck, or beef, to bison, lamb, pork, or fish. It is best to use bones from locally sourced meat that was grass-fed or pasture-raised, or sustainable, wild-caught salt-water fish. Once the broth is made, it can be consumed on its own or used in the preparation of other dishes as a building block for soups, stews, grains, or bean dishes.

The following basic bone broth recipes are for making bone broth at home. The size of the pot considered best for the basic broth recipes is an 18 quart stockpot. We recommend using stainless steel stockpots or cast-iron pots. Please note that most large cast-iron pots hold 9 quarts, and if you choose to use them, you may reduce the amount of bones by 2–3 pounds in the recipes, or one fewer whole fish. For those who are not comfortable simmering broth on the stove for the length of time it takes to make bone broth, slow cookers are an alternative. However, most slow cookers are smaller than the suggested pots—the largest we found on the market were 8 quart slow cookers. If you choose to use a slow cooker, it is best to follow the ratio adjusted for a cast-iron pot.

The amount of bones and the type of bones suggested in our basic broth recipes produce the richest, most gelatinous broths. Gelatinous broths are the most beneficial for digestive health. However, even if you don't have the full amount or type of bones indicated (for example, if you only have marrow and less-cartilage-rich beef bones), your broth will still be flavorful, nutritious, and beneficial to your health. Fish broth is not naturally very high in gelatin content. The good news is that fish broth offers iodine, a unique nutrient not present in the other animal bone broths.

Though the lengthy process of making bone broth is mostly passive work, we strongly recommend that you check the pot along the way to ensure just a bare simmer throughout the whole cooking time. You want to avoid holding the broth at a rolling boil and also avoid too low of a temperature. Ideally, you will be able to see tiny bubbles gently appearing and disappearing. We find that it is easier to maintain the desired temperature by keeping the lid off the pot or slightly tilted, half-covering the pot. Also, skim any scum that rises to the surface for a cleaner and better-tasting broth.

Please note that all of these broths can be made simply with a combination of bones and water only. We like to add apple cider vinegar to optimize the extraction of minerals from the bones. Some people are sensitive to vinegar. The omission of vinegar will still produce a potent and nutritious broth. The added ingredients for each type of broth are suggestions from the recipes that we use at our company and at home, and that we enjoy for the flavor they impart and for how they complement the inherent flavor and energy of each type of bone.

TIP FOR KEEPING ENOUGH BONES IN YOUR HOME STOCK

Beef, lamb, pork, and bison bones are easier to source from your butcher than chicken, turkey, duck, and fish bones might be. Small local butchers and fishmongers often sell the whole animals, not the bones separately. There are great benefits to purchasing whole animals. Not only is it cheaper, but the various parts of the whole animal provide unique nutritional value, and when consumed in collaboration provide complete nutrition. Every time that you roast, poach, or bake a chicken, turkey, or fish at home, keep the bones! Just store them in a freezer-safe container or bag. Alternatively, ask your farmer or butcher to set some bones aside for you to pick up when available. If you want to make the most gelatinous broth, consider requesting feet. Feet in general provide abundant cartilage, and adding chicken, pork, or calves' feet will make your broth wonderfully gelatinous.

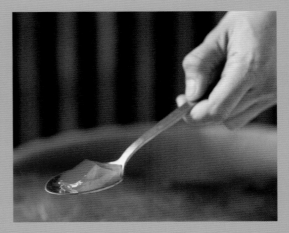

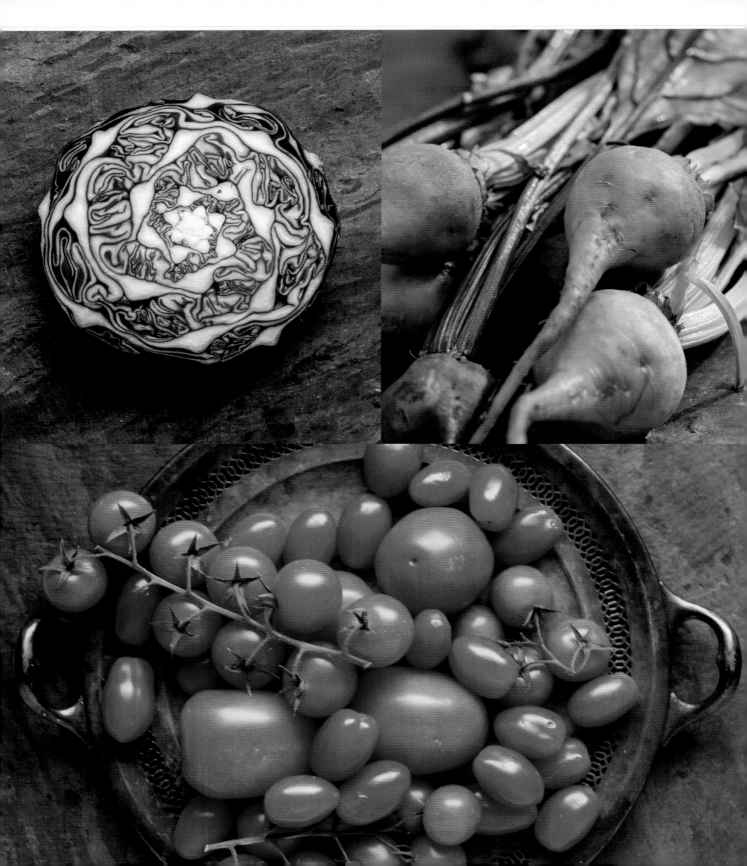

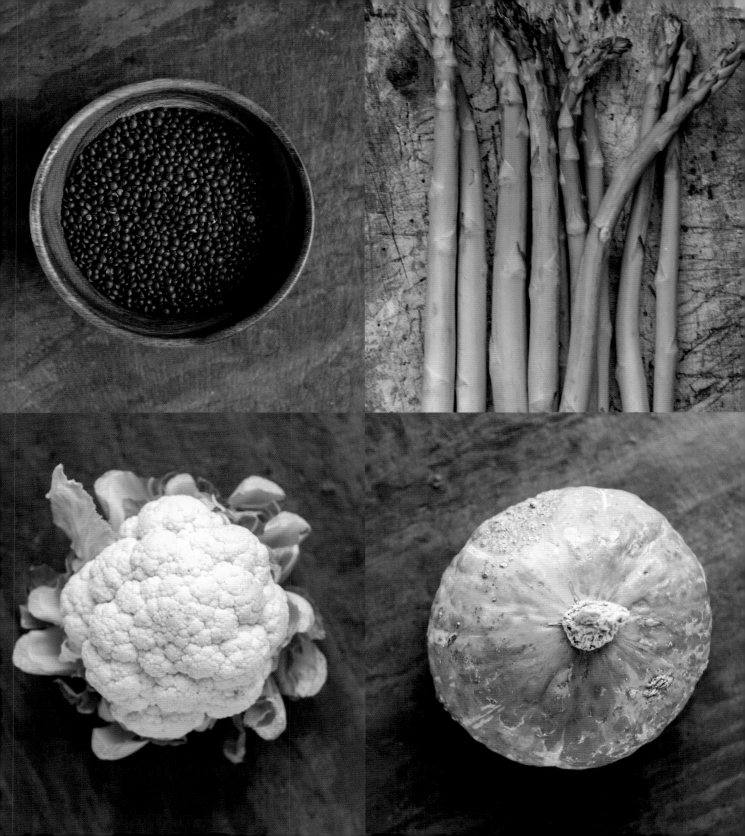

adds to your dishes. While ginger does come fresh or ground, the flavor of each is quite different, so be careful substituting! We love it in a basic beef bone broth preparation.

FRESH FENNEL

Fennel is used for indigestion, spasms in the digestive tract, and expelling phlegm from the lungs. Fennel is rich with the antioxidant flavonoid quercetin, known for its anti-inflammatory effects, as a natural antihistamine, and as useful for helping reduce blood pressure.

GARLIC

Alliums have a great flavor range from their raw state to cooked. The pungency and flavor of raw garlic that give a bang to fresh pestos and dressings transform to a savory caramelized sweetness when roasted. Garlic has plenty of antioxidants and is known to be a natural blood thinner.

ONION

Onion is a basic but versatile ingredient with many varieties, from shallots to vidalia to red onions, each imparting a unique flavor. To boot, the skins contain almost double the antioxidants of the onion itself, as well as additional quercetin. Although the skin is not edible, the benefits can be reaped by adding it to your broths and removing it before serving.

BASIL

Basil and other leafy green herbs are best added in the final moments of cooking or used as a garnish to maintain their bright color and fresh flavor. Basil is rich in vitamin A, which is important for retina health. Experiment with different basil varieties like lemon or Thai basil. Basil is great in our Vietnamese Pho (p. 49), Yellow Thai Curry (p. 135), and Malaysian Laksa (p. 142).

CILANTRO

Aside from being a delicious addition and finishing touch to anything from salsas and ceviches to soups, cilantro is cited as being useful for detoxification from heavy metals and as a natural cleansing agent. Cilantro also contains abundant levels of vitamins A, C, and K. Try it in Pozole with Garbanzo Beans in Tomatillo and Pumpkin Seed Broth (p. 94), Spicy Prawn Stew (p. 141), Vietnamese Pho (p. 49), and Yellow Thai Curry (p. 135).

PARSLEY

Some may think of parsley as the plain Jane of green herbs, but its simple, clean flavor makes it a versatile addition to a variety of recipes. Parsley is rich in vitamins A, B12, K, and C. It also supports kidney function by flushing excess fluid from the body. It is a great addition to the basic broth recipes—just make sure you add it during the last 15 minutes of cooking to retain its nutrients. Try it in our Quinoa and Artichoke Salad with Lemon, Capers, Parsley, and Thyme (p. 82) and in any of our soup recipes.

DILL

Dill's feathery fronds offer a distinct flavor that we enjoy best with chicken. Try it as a garnish in our Tequila Consommé or with fish and spring flavors such as carrots, peas, and cucumbers. A little goes a long way!

SEAWEEDS

Seaweeds qualify as a superfood in our book. The many different varieties of seaweeds offer blood purifying, alkalizing, and detoxifying properties, while giving a generous boost of minerals, specifically iodine and calcium. As with sourcing your meats and seafood, be sure you are buying clean and quality seaweeds. Seaweeds will absorb the properties of the water in which they are grown, so you want to ensure that they have been grown and harvested in unpolluted waters that are pure and free from harmful chemicals.

Dulse and nori are nice when flaked and added as seasonings to a final dish, or as snacks on their own. Other varieties, such as kelp, kombu, and arame, provide interesting texture and subtle salty minerality to simple broths. Asian cultures, in fact, often prescribe seaweed soups for healing and recovery postpartum. Remember, though, dried seaweeds will expand a generous amount when rehydrated! Try them in the Seafood Miso Soup recipe (p. 132).

VINEGAR

There are tons of varieties of vinegar, but for our broth-making purposes, we most often use apple cider vinegar. Adding apple cider vinegar to your broth helps to extract more mineral content from the bones. Taken on its own, apple cider vinegar is useful for alleviating leg cramps at night, balancing the pH of your skin, supporting the liver's detoxification mechanisms, breaking up mucus in the body, moving lymph, and stimulating digestion.

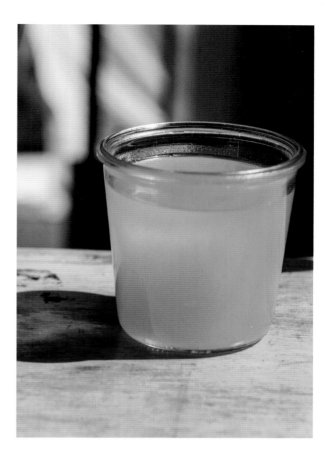

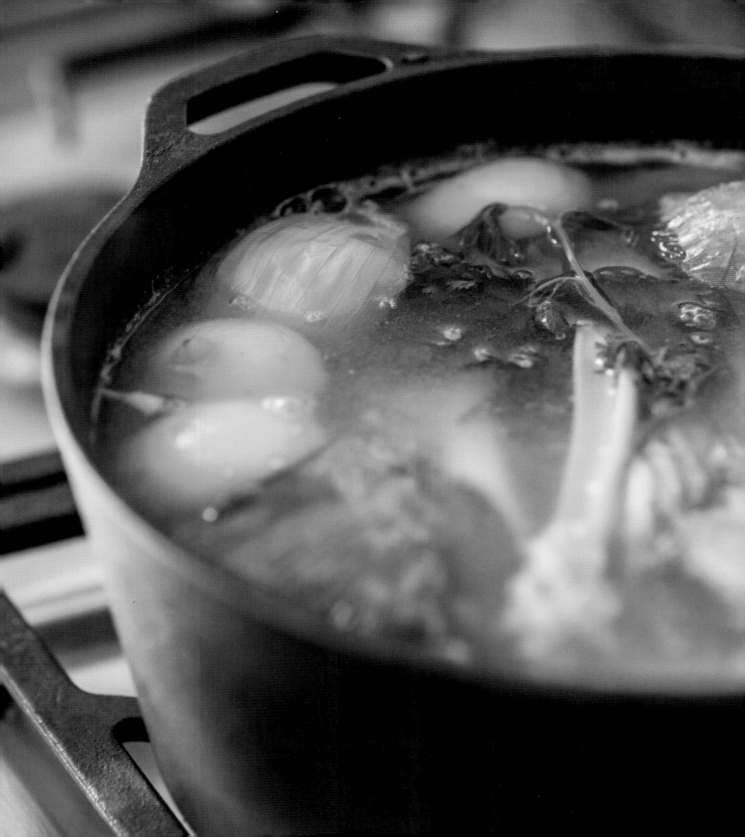

Equipment

THOUGH ALUMINUM IS LIGHTWEIGHT AND CHEAP, it is highly reactive to acidic and alkaline foods, causing the metal to leach into your food, especially when the metal is not properly cared for. Aluminum is a soft metal and therefore easily scratched and warped. It is also commonly treated with questionable nonstick finishes. Stainless steel, on the other hand, is more durable and doesn't react with food while still being affordable.

We also love cast iron. Our cast-iron pots and pans require a little more energy to maintain, but we say it's worth it. Yes, they're heavy, but plain cast-iron has unparalleled heat capacity and durability and is naturally nonstick (and just think of those cut arms you'll be flaunting after all your cast-iron cooking!). The thickness of cast-iron pots and pans also results in even heating and requires just a little extra time to heat up. Cooking with cast iron also contributes iron as a nutrient to the food. All of these benefits, though, come from well-cared-for and seasoned cast-iron, so be sure to take the extra few minutes to wash your cast-iron pots with water and reseason them often.

USEFUL TOOLS

* Stainless-steel pots or cast-iron pots, enameled or not. Our recipes call for 18 quart pots, and we recommend that you invest in a pot of this size or larger to make larger batches at a time.
* Large kitchen tongs
* Spider skimmers (skimmers with a long handle and a web-like design) or slotted spoons
* Large colander
* Large containers to hold the strained broth for cooling
* Freezer-safe wide-mouth glass jars, pint and quart sizes, or food-grade BPA-free plastic for freezer storage
* Labels
* Permanent marker

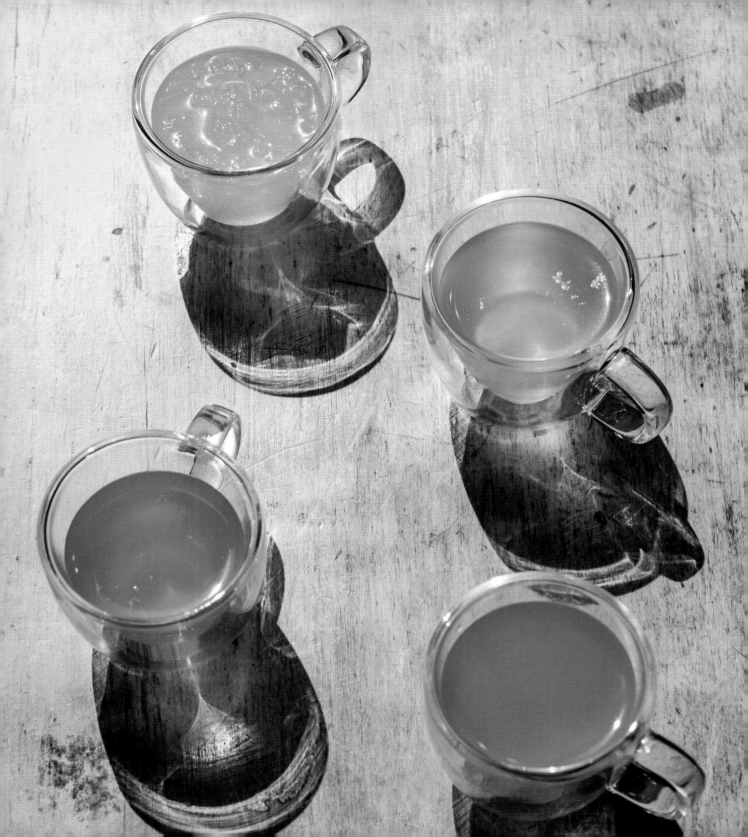

Basic Broths

ALL OF THE FOLLOWING RECIPES CAN BE MADE with a combination of bones and water only. Each one includes an optional list of ingredients, adding vinegar for maximum mineral extraction from the bones, and aromatics that we find complement the flavor of the bones of each type of animal. Feel free to combine bones from similar animals. For example, make broth from any combination of beef, lamb, and bison bones or chicken, turkey, and duck. We prefer to combine fish bones only with different types of fish or shellfish. Broth made from pig's feet and hocks is very gelatinous and neutral tasting. Pig's feet and hocks can be combined with any other type of bones, especially if you have few bones available or if you don't have bones that are rich in cartilage and connective tissue.

For a very special and very rich-tasting broth, we recommend a double broth. First make a basic bone broth with aromatics. Strain, cool, and skim the broth. Then, with fresh roasted or cleaned bones and fresh aromatics, make the double broth by using the previous broth as the liquid base for the new broth.

These recipes will serve as your guides, but they are not set in stone. Use the amount of bones that is available to you, even if it is not the exact amount presented here. Just make sure that when you add water, you add only enough to barely cover the bones.

BONE MEAL

If after making broth you end up with very soft bones, there is more to do with them than just giving them to your dog! You can grind them to make bone meal. We learned this from Vlasta, a photographer we met when we were being interviewed for a feature on Bone Deep & Harmony. Vlasta was born in Russia, and she shared with us that her grandmother was in the habit of making and eating bone meal—a common practice where she grew up.

To make bone meal, clean the bones after making bone broth, removing meat and any fat from the bones. Roast the bones at 400°F for 1 hour or until they become very dry and brittle. Allow them to cool a little and place them in a sack made of a firm cloth. Pound the bones to break into small pieces. You may use a meat tenderizer or a small hammer. Transfer to a food processor or a blender and grind into bone meal.

Vlasta told us that once the bone meal was ground, it would be added into the broth. Admittedly, we have yet to try this, but there is no question that it would be the most potent calcium-providing soup! Bone meal may also be used as a nourishing organic plant fertilizer.

Beef or Bison Bone Broth

A COMBINATION OF KNUCKLE AND/OR THIGHBONES AND MARROWBONES
makes the best broth. Knucklebones produce the most gelatinous broth.
Add a few meaty bones from the shanks or oxtails for the most delicious broth.

Yield: About 8 quarts

10–12 pounds beef or bison bones

Water

OPTIONAL

1 bunch scallions, cleaned

1 large onion, quartered

1 head garlic

1 thumb-sized piece ginger root, sliced

¼ cup apple cider vinegar

4 teaspoons salt

1. Roast or clean the bones. Roasting the bones imparts depth of flavor and color to the broth. Cleaning the bones gives the broth a cleaner taste and mouthfeel. To roast the bones, place them in a 400°F oven for 45–60 minutes or until the bones are golden brown, turning the bones once during this time. Discard the fat released from the bones and proceed with the basic recipe. If you do not roast the bones, you must clean them first to prevent your final broth from developing an off taste. Simply cover the bones with cold water, bring to a boil, and lower the heat to simmer them for 10 minutes. Discard the water and proceed with the basic recipe.

2. Place the roasted or cleaned bones in the pot and cover with cold water, barely covering the bones. Bring the water to a boil and reduce the heat immediately, to as low as possible while maintaining a bare simmer. You should be able to see tiny bubbles. Add the optional ingredients at this point, if using.

3. Leave the broth simmering for at least 12 hours and up to 24 hours. The longer you simmer it, the more nutrition will be extracted from the bones. Check on your broth every now and again during this time to ensure that the temperature at which you are simmering remains constant, and that the water level still covers the bones. Add more water as necessary. When the broth is ready, turn off the heat and allow the broth to cool thoroughly before straining. Depending on the size of the pot you used, it will take a few hours to come down to room temperature.

4. When the broth is cool in the pot, remove the bones first. We use tongs and a spider skimmer. Set the bones aside. Strain and transfer the broth to one large container to refrigerate before skimming or to the individual containers you will use for final storage. Pull out any salvageable meat from what was strained out of the broth and discard all other ingredients. Refrigerate the strained broth for a few hours until it thickens and all the fat congeals on the top.

5. You may keep the layer of fat for longer storage, as it seals the broth effectively from oxygen, which could spoil the broth quicker. Or you may skim the broth at this time. Poke through the fat with a paring knife, lift it, and pick the fat up with your hands. Discard the fat or save it for another use (see the section on tallow, p. 153). If you used a large container to refrigerate the broth before skimming, you may now transfer the skimmed broth to individual containers for storage. Label and date each container. Skimmed broth lasts up to 1 week in the refrigerator and 6 months in the freezer.

WHAT TO DO WITH YOUR LEFTOVER BONES

Sometimes at the end of cooking you may find there is a little marrow left in the bones. You can usually rescue this nutrient-dense goodness by tapping the bones to release the soft marrow from the fibrous matrix. The remaining marrow can be added to baby foods or soups, added to your mug of broth, used as a spread on toast, or enjoyed as a delicious treat on its own. You may also find some meat left on the bones or in the bowl of strained ingredients. This meat is super tender after a long, slow simmer and is also a great snack, or it may be added back into your broth or soup. We sometimes add a little seasoning and stick it back in the oven on the lowest temperature to dehydrate it for our own homemade jerky. Last, if the bones are still dense, you may keep them in the freezer and reuse them in your next batch along with fresh bones for more gelatin and nutrients.

Lamb or Goat Bone Broth

FROM A TRADITIONAL CHINESE MEDICINE PERSPECTIVE, CONSUMING THE MEAT AND bones of lamb and goat has the most warming effect in the body. For that reason, it is not necessary to use too many of these bones when making broth. When we make lamb broth using a ratio of fewer bones to water, we normally end up with a clearer and less gelatinous broth. Sometimes, we just add a couple lamb bones to beef or bison bone broth. Our favorite aromatics with this warming broth include cinnamon, cardamom, and turmeric root.

Yield: About 4 quarts

3–5 pounds lamb or goat bones

Water

OPTIONAL

1 onion, quartered

3 cloves garlic, smashed

3 cardamom pods

1 inch piece fresh turmeric root or ginger root

1 cinnamon stick

1 bay leaf

2 teaspoons salt

1. Roast or clean the bones as indicated in the Beef or Bison Bone Broth recipe (p. 30).

2. Pour cold water over the roasted or cleaned bones to cover. For this broth, you may use more water than with other broths, leaving a couple of inches below the rim of the pot.

3. Bring to a boil and reduce the heat immediately to hold the water at a bare simmer.

4. Add the optional ingredients, if using. Simmer for 12 hours.

5. Turn off the heat and let the broth cool down, in the pot, to room temperature.

6. Strain the broth, discard the solids, and transfer the broth to a large container or the final smaller containers you will use for storage. Refrigerate for several hours or overnight.

7. Skim the broth. This broth will have less fat than the beef broth. Pour it into your choice of storage containers if you have not yet done so. Label and date your containers. Keep in the refrigerator for up to 1 week or freeze for up to 6 months.

Chicken, Turkey, or Duck Bone Broth

CHICKEN BONE BROTH IS PROBABLY THE MOST ACCESSIBLE START FOR FOLKS
who are new to making bone broth. It is culturally familiar, and the smaller
size of the bones makes it easier to prepare.

In Chinese medicine, it is believed that the energy of the birds is concentrated in the skin.
A practical and delicious way to prepare broth is to start with a whole chicken, and to poach it for
1 hour before removing it from the pot to pick the meat off the bones. Reserve the meat for other
meals, and return the bones back into the pot to continue simmering for bone broth. Save the bones
from previous meals of roast chicken, turkey, or duck in your freezer, and add those to your next pot
of broth. One more tip: the feet, necks and heads of birds make the most gelatinous broths!

Yield: About 8 quarts

10 pounds chicken, turkey, or
duck bones (or a combination),
preferably including necks and
chicken feet

Water

OPTIONAL

2 onions, quartered

2 celery stalks, roughly chopped

3 carrots, roughly chopped

1 head garlic, smashed

1 tablespoon fennel seeds

1 tablespoon coriander seeds

½ tablespoon peppercorns

2 bay leaves

A few sprigs herbs, such as thyme,
sage, or rosemary

2 tablespoons apple cider vinegar

4 teaspoons salt

1. If you are using the bones from previously cooked chicken, turkey, or duck, you don't have to clean or roast the bones. If you start with raw bones, cover the bones in cold water, bring to a boil, and simmer at medium heat for about 10 minutes.

2. Discard the water and fill the pot with cold water again to barely cover the bones. Bring to a boil and reduce the heat immediately. Add the optional ingredients, if using.

3. Simmer for 8–12 hours. Turn off the heat and let the broth come to room temperature in the pot.

4. Strain and transfer to a large container or to individual storage containers. Refrigerate for several hours or overnight. The fat will congeal on the top. Chicken, turkey, and duck fat does not solidify as much as beef fat. You will need a slotted spoon to skim the fat off.

5. Label and date the containers and refrigerate for 1 week or freeze for up to 6 months.

Pork Bone Broth

PORK BONES ARE VERY RICH IN CARTILAGE AND COLLAGEN, AND YOU MAY USE FEWER BONES to produce an equally gelatinous broth. We recommend the feet and hocks. We fell in love with pork broth when we started working with it. It is the most neutral tasting of all the broths we make, and it can be used interchangeably with any of the recipes we present in this book.

Yield: About 4 quarts

5–7 pounds pork feet (split) and hocks

Water

OPTIONAL

1 head garlic

2 tablespoons apple cider vinegar

2 teaspoons salt

1. Start by cleaning the bones. Cover with cold water, bring the water to a boil, then reduce the heat and simmer for 10 minutes.

2. Strain and discard the water and return the bones to the pot with enough fresh water to barely cover the bones. Bring to a boil and then reduce the heat to a bare simmer. Add the optional ingredients, if using, and simmer for 8 hours.

3. Cool the broth in the pot to room temperature, then strain it into a large container or your choice of storage containers. Refrigerate for several hours.

4. Skim the layer of fat that congeals on the top. If you have not done so yet, pour the broth into storage containers. Label and date your containers. Leave in the refrigerator for 1 week or freeze for up to 6 months.

Fish Bone Broth

THE COLLAGEN IN FISH BROTH IS NOT AS TIGHTLY BOUND AS THAT IN THE BONES OF BIRDS
and mammals, which is why fish bones dissolve more quickly. Fish bone broth can be made in
1 hour! In the United States, most people are not in the habit of purchasing and cooking whole fish,
but we recommend doing so for your broth making. If you buy a whole fish, roast it, fry it,
or bake it; eat the flesh; and keep the bones and heads to make fish broth. Including fish heads in
your broth produces a nutritious iodine-rich and thyroid-supporting broth. We love fish broth
especially during the warmer months because it is lighter and it pairs so well with fresh herbs.
The added seaweed in the optional ingredients provides an extra boost of sea minerals.

Yield: About 4 quarts

1 tablespoon butter

1 onion, chopped

2 carrots, chopped

1 stalk celery, chopped

1 bulb fennel, chopped

1 cup white wine

Bones and heads of 3 medium white-flesh fish, washed (oily fish do not produce a good-tasting broth, and the oils may become rancid during cooking)

Water

5 sprigs thyme

1 lemon, sliced

2 tablespoons apple cider vinegar

2 teaspoons salt

1 4-inch piece kombu or kelp seaweed

1. Melt the butter in a stockpot over medium heat. Add the onion, carrots, celery, and fennel. Mix the vegetables well and let them sweat until they soften.

2. Increase the heat and add the wine. After a few minutes, add the fish bones and heads and cover with a little more than 4 quarts cold water. Bring the water to a simmer, then reduce the heat to low. Add the thyme, lemon, vinegar, and salt. Gently simmer for at least 1 hour and up to 4 hours.

3. Add the seaweed, if using, during the last 15 minutes of cooking.

4. Turn off the heat and allow the broth to cool thoroughly.

5. Strain the broth and discard all solids. Store in the refrigerator for 1 week or in the freezer for up to 6 months.

Making Bone Broth in the Slow Cooker

MANY PEOPLE FEEL UNDERSTANDABLY UNEASY ABOUT LEAVING THE STOVE ON FOR THE length of time that bone broth preparation requires. An alternative is to use a slow cooker. Slow cookers are smaller than stockpots, with the larger ones yielding about 4 quarts of broth. Although this method is perfectly practical, we prefer the flavor achieved with the broth simmering over fire. If you choose to use a slow cooker, here is a basic guideline recipe. You may use any bones or combination of bones.

Yield: About 4 quarts

Beef or bison bones: about 5–7 pounds, simmer for 24 hours

Lamb or goat bones: 3–4 pounds, simmer for 12 hours

Chicken, turkey, or duck bones: 3–4 pounds, simmer for 8–12 hours

Pork bones: 2 pig's feet (split) and 1 or 2 hocks, simmer for 8–12 hours

Fish: the bones and heads of 2 or 3 medium fish, simmer for 1–4 hours

2 tablespoons apple cider vinegar

OPTIONAL

Aromatics such as 1 carrot, chopped; 1 stalk celery, chopped; 4 cloves garlic, smashed; 1 onion, quartered; 1 thumb-sized piece ginger root, chopped; 1 bouquet garni

1. Place your chosen bones in the slow cooker and add cold water to barely cover. Add the apple cider vinegar and let stand for 30–60 minutes.

2. Add any aromatics, if using. Cover, and set the cooker on low. Cook for the amount of time indicated for each type of bone. Check the slow cooker a few times along the way, adding water if necessary. Also, skim off any scum that rises to the surface.

3. Turn off the slow cooker and let the broth cool to room temperature.

4. Remove the bones with tongs and a spider skimmer or slotted spoon. Strain and transfer the broth to a large container or several smaller storage containers. Refrigerate for several hours or overnight.

5. Skim the fat off, and if you have not yet done so, pour the broth into individual storage containers. Label and date your containers. Refrigerate for up to 1 week or freeze for up to 6 months.

TIPS FOR MAKING YOUR BROTH GEL

- Use bones that have the most cartilage and connective tissue. Some examples are knucklebones, necks, and feet.

- If you are lucky enough to find Achilles tendons, these will undoubtedly yield a gelatinous broth.

- The amount of water you use can be a determining factor of how gelatinous your broth will end up being. Add enough water to barely cover the bones for best results. Check your broth constantly to maintain the same level of water, adding more if necessary.

- Make sure that the temperature at which your broth simmers is as low as possible but still produces tiny bubbles, and that it remains constant. If the temperature is too high, the collagen may be broken down too much, making it unable to coagulate when you cool the broth.

STORING YOUR BROTH

The best option for storing your broth is in freezer-safe glass jars. The classic pint-sized Mason jars are convenient for 1–2 servings and quick to defrost. Be sure to buy the freezer-safe wide-mouth jars and reserve about an inch of space at the top to allow the broth to expand upon freezing. It is also important to refrigerate the broth before freezing. A fine alternative to glass is BPA-free plastic, which comes in a wider variety of shapes and sizes and can be more convenient for maximizing freezer space. We also like using ice cube trays to make broth cubes. These are great for recipes that call for just a small amount of broth, when cooking for just one, or for storing your double broth or broth-based sauces.

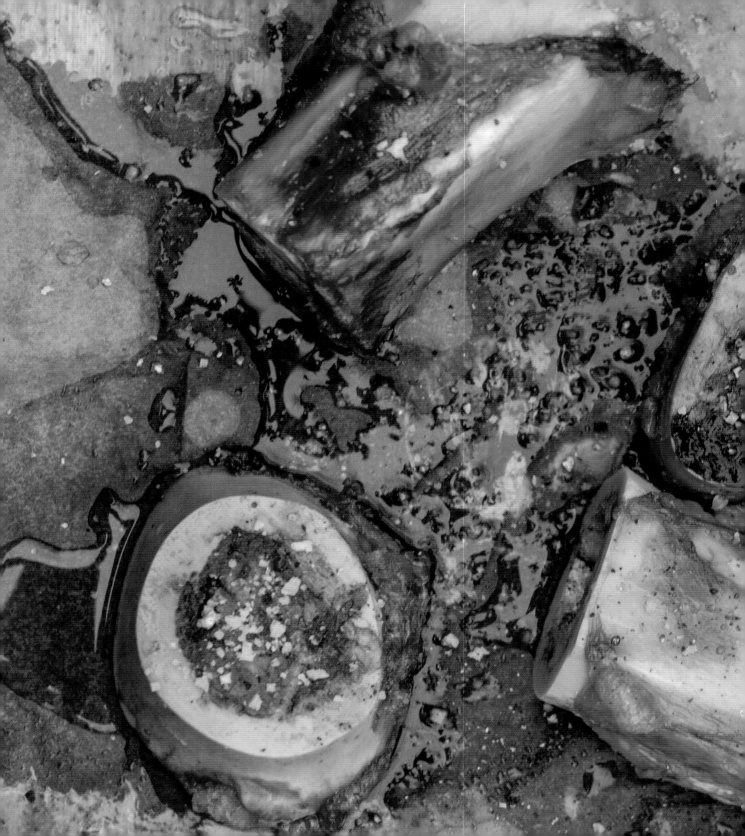

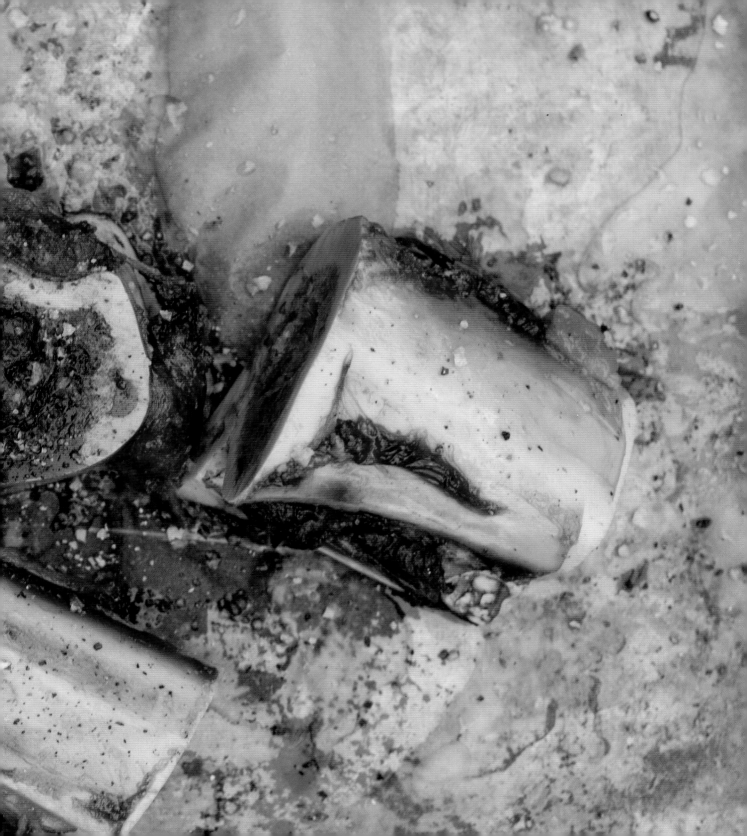

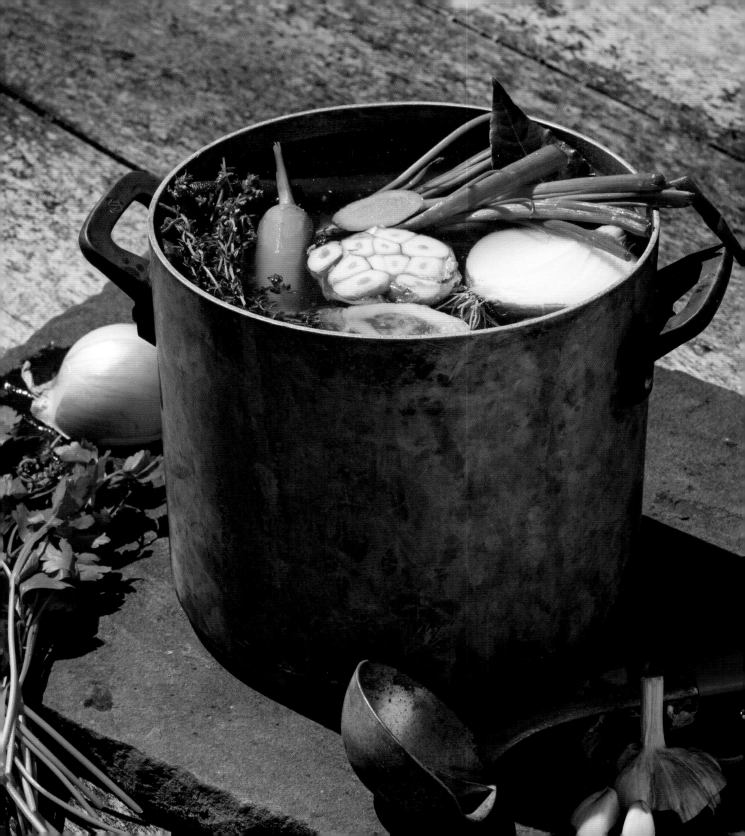

Recipes

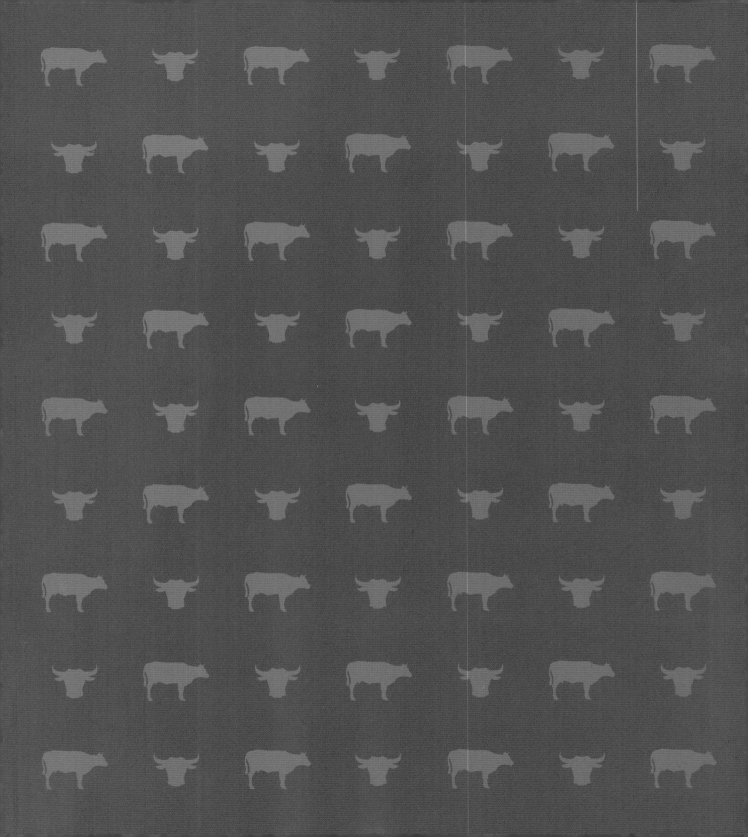

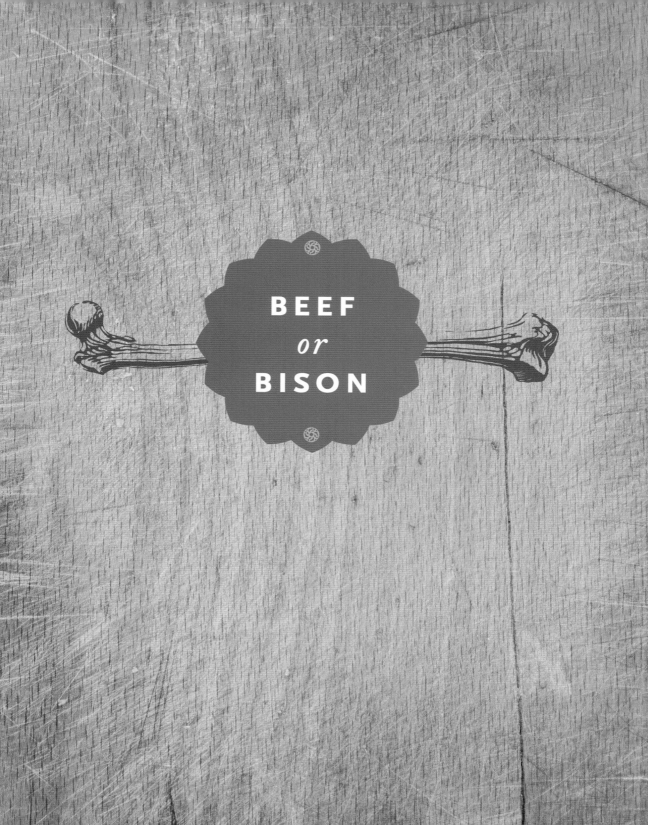

BEEF

or

BISON

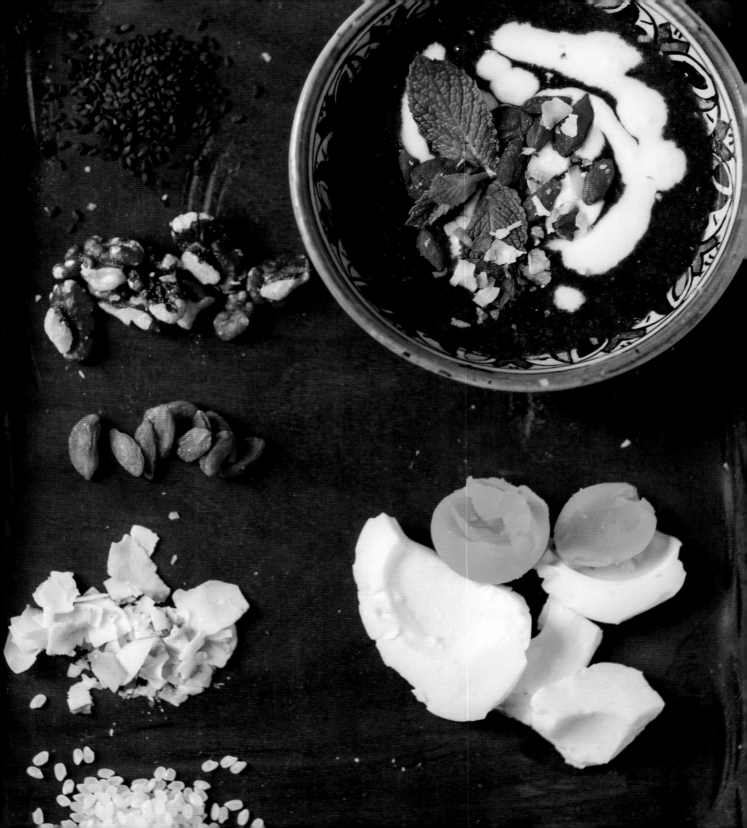

Black Sesame and Jujube Jook with Coconut Milk

JUJUBES ARE A VARIETY OF DATES COMMONLY USED IN KOREAN COOKING THAT YOU CAN FIND at most Asian supermarkets or herbal pharmacies, but any dried fruit will work. We often substitute mulberries, gojis, medjool dates, dried tart cherries, cranberries, or figs.

Yield: 6 servings

1 cup sweet sticky rice

½ cup black sesame seeds

2 cups filtered water, divided use

3 cups beef bone broth

½ cup dried jujube dates, pitted and chopped

½ tablespoon maple syrup + additional to taste

½ cup full-fat coconut milk

Maldon flaky sea salt

Fresh mint

Toasted coconut

Pine nuts

1. Soak the rice in water overnight. Rinse and drain.

2. Rinse and drain the black sesame seeds. Finely grind the rice with 1 cup water. Set aside.

3. Blend the black sesame seeds with the remaining water, starting with less water and gradually adding more. If you have a rice cooker, mix the blended rice and black sesame seeds with the broth and dates in the rice cooker and cook on the setting for glutinous rice.

4. If cooking on the stove, add the liquid rice and sesame mixture and dates to a large pot, turn the heat to medium-high, and stir until it starts to boil. Stir in the broth. Cook at low heat for 10–15 minutes. Continue to stir to prevent any rice from sticking to the bottom of the pot.

5. When the jook is fully cooked, it should be quite thick (the consistency of thick batter). You can always thin it by adding additional water or broth, or thicken it by cooking for a few extra minutes.

6. Mix the maple syrup with coconut milk to your desired sweetness.

7. Serve the porridge in bowls topped with a pinch of flaky salt, like Maldon, a generous drizzle of the sweetened coconut milk, a few sprigs of fresh mint, toasted coconut, and pine nuts.

Gingered Borscht

THIS RECIPE FOR THE TRADITIONAL RUSSIAN BEET SOUP IS SPICED UP WITH CUMIN, GINGER, and bay leaves. We also add apple, carrots, and red bell pepper. It is delicious with a sprinkling of fresh dill, a dollop of sheep's milk yogurt, and a small spoonful of wild salmon roe. A simple soup, for sure, but its crimson velvety look and feel, topped with the bright pink salmon roe, give it enough character to be served alone or as a main dish. Paired with a piece of crusty sourdough bread, it makes a perfect snowy weather meal!

Yield: 4–6 servings

1 tablespoon butter (preferably grass-fed and cultured, raw if possible)

1 tablespoon extra virgin olive oil

1 large onion, diced

3 large beets, peeled and diced

2 carrots, diced

1 red bell pepper, cored and diced

1 apple, cored and diced

1 thumb-sized piece ginger root, peeled and finely chopped

1 teaspoon cumin seeds, lightly toasted

1 bay leaf

6 cups beef bone broth, divided use

Salt

GARNISHES (OPTIONAL)

Fresh sprigs dill

Sheep or goat milk yogurt

Wild salmon roe

1. In a large, heavy-bottomed pot, melt the butter and olive oil. Add the onion.

2. When the onion is soft, add the beets, carrots, bell pepper, apple, ginger, cumin seeds, bay leaf, and 1 cup broth. Mix all the vegetables and aromatics thoroughly. Half-cover the pot and allow the vegetables to sweat.

3. After about 10 minutes, add the remaining 5 cups broth to the pot. Bring to a boil and reduce the heat. Simmer gently for about 30 minutes. Turn off the heat.

4. Once the soup is cool enough to handle, blend most of the vegetables, leaving some in the pot, with some of the cooking liquid, using an immersion blender, food processor, or regular blender. Return the blended portion of the soup to the pot. Mix well, salt to taste, and return the soup to a simmer.

5. Once the soup is warm, pour into bowls and top each bowl with a dollop of yogurt, a sprinkling of dill, and a small spoonful of roe.

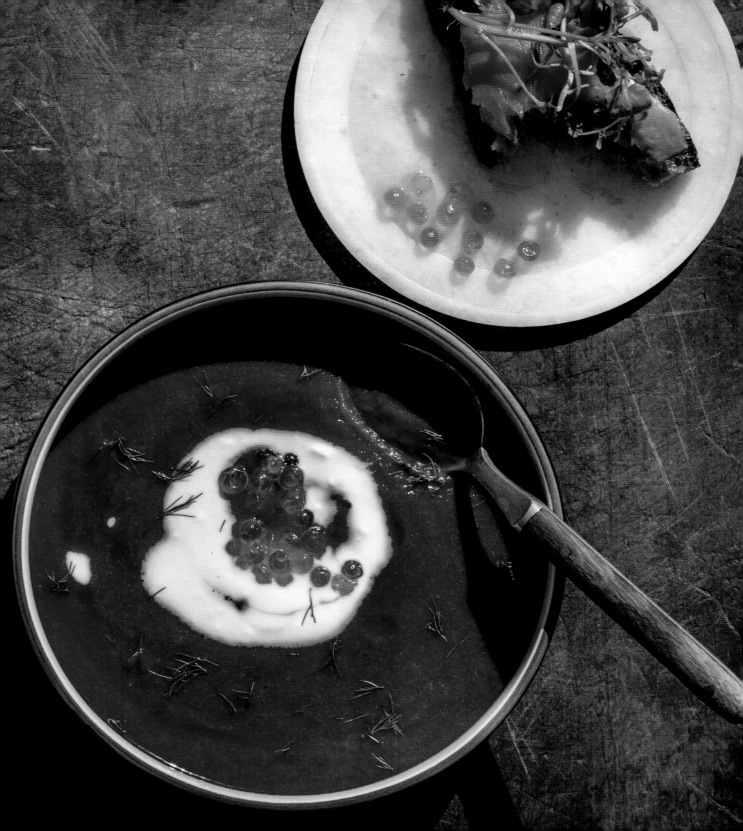

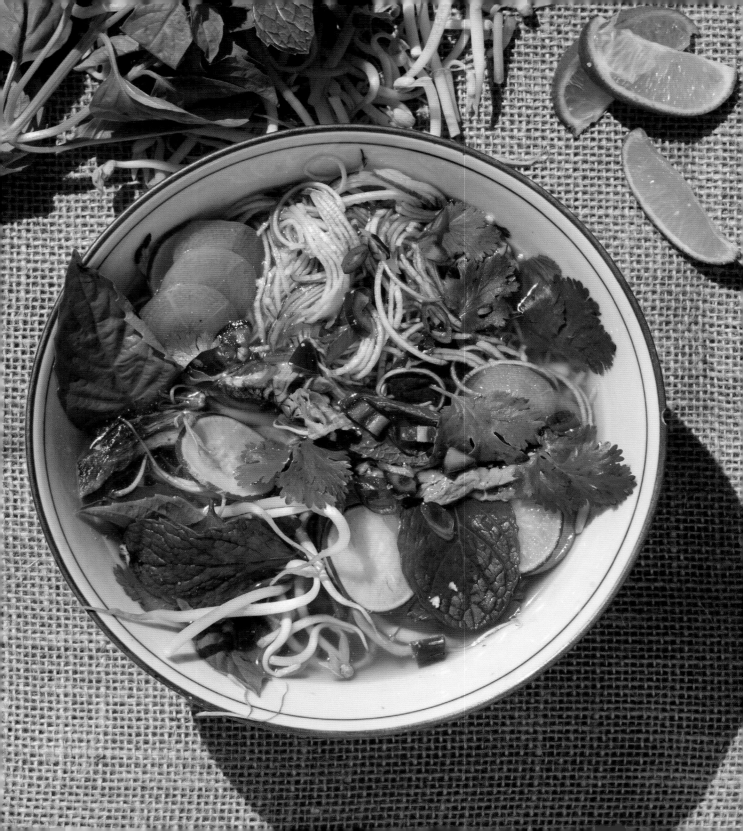

Vietnamese Pho

OUR FAMILIES LOVE PHO. WE LIKE IT AS MUCH IN THE WINTER AS IN THE SUMMER.
On warm days, we enjoy it garnished with plenty of fresh herbs and thinly sliced raw vegetables.
During cooler months, we have it with hearty cooked vegetables, and buckwheat noodles or rice.
Add any vegetables and condiments that you fancy to make your own version.

Yield: 4–6 servings

2 quarts beef bone broth

1 star anise

1 small cinnamon stick

½ teaspoon coriander seeds

½ teaspoon fennel seeds

¼ teaspoon whole cloves

6 cardamom pods

2 tablespoons nama shoyu or tamari (soy sauce)

1 tablespoon fish sauce

2 teaspoons coconut sugar

Salt and pepper

1 zucchini, spiral sliced, or your choice of noodles or cooked rice

½ pound fresh bean sprouts

1 small raw steak, thinly sliced

GARNISH

Mint

Cilantro

Basil sprigs

Scallions, slivered

2 fresh chiles, such as jalapeños or serranos, thinly sliced

Lime wedges

1. Bring the broth to a boil and turn down the heat to a simmer. Add the star anise, cinnamon, coriander, fennel, cloves, and cardamom. Add shoyu or tamari, fish sauce, coconut sugar, and salt and pepper to taste. Simmer, covered, for 30 minutes. Taste for salt and add more if necessary.

2. Strain the broth. At this point, the broth may be refrigerated to serve later; simply heat it to piping hot before serving.

3. When ready to serve the pho, place a handful of the zucchini slices or your choice of noodles or rice in each bowl. Top with some bean sprouts and a few slices of the raw steak. Ladle hot broth over the raw meat into the bowls. The meat will cook in the broth very quickly, especially the more thinly it is sliced. Serve with a large platter of the garnishes to pass for everyone to add to their liking.

Spicy Carrot Soup

A SIMPLE CARROT SOUP IS A QUICK AND EASY RECIPE TO ADD TO YOUR BROTH-BASED SOUP rotation. This one contains loads of ginger for its cleansing and stimulating properties. We eat this simple soup year round, sometimes adding coconut milk or spices like cumin or curry for a winter version, or serving it chilled or room temperature with loads of fresh herbs or pea shoots in the spring and summer. Aside from the broth, this is an otherwise vegan recipe and a great introductory dish for any friends who may be a little squeamish about bone broth. Our kids eat it up, too!

Yield: 8 servings

2 tablespoons coconut oil

2 onions, peeled and chopped

6 cups chicken or beef bone broth

2 pounds carrots, peeled and sliced

3 tablespoons grated fresh ginger root

OPTIONAL

1 cup organic unsweetened full-fat coconut milk (if using coconut milk, reduce the amount of broth by 1 cup)

Fresh herbs, such as parsley, dill, or cilantro

Fresh pesto

Toasted pumpkin seeds

1. Heat the coconut oil in a saucepan over medium heat. Add the onions and cook until soft.

2. Add the broth, carrots, and ginger. Reduce the heat to a simmer and cook until the carrots are tender when pierced.

3. Remove the soup from the heat and allow it to rest for 5 minutes. Pour it into a blender in batches and pulse to start, then purée until smooth. When making this or any blended soup, save yourself from learning the hard way or splatter-painting your kitchen walls by covering the top of the blender with a dish cloth and holding it down extra tight. It's also a good idea not to overfill the blender and to blend in batches.

4. Return the blended soup to the pot. Stir in the coconut milk (if using) and heat to a simmer.

5. Serve garnished with herbs, pesto, or pumpkin seeds, as desired.

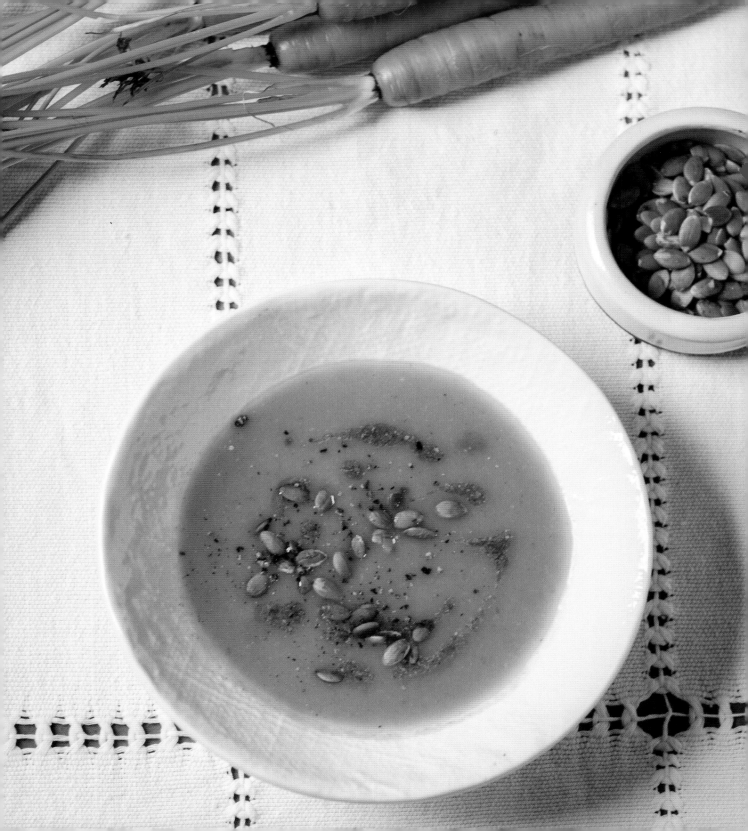

Black Garlic and Roasted Bone Marrow Soup with Crispy Herbs

IN TAOIST MYTHOLOGY, BLACK GARLIC IS RUMORED TO GRANT IMMORTALITY. WE CAN'T PROMISE YOU that, but there's no doubt that black garlic is great for your health—it's loaded with nearly twice as many antioxidants as raw garlic. In combination with nutrient-dense bone marrow and broth, you might just call this a superfood soup! Black garlic is most commonly found at Asian or Italian markets. It has a sweet/savory flavor, molasses-like color, and tender texture. It's a great secret ingredient!

Yield: 4 servings

4 pounds marrowbones

3 tablespoons olive oil, divided use

½ teaspoon sea salt + additional to taste

3 tablespoons butter

2 shallots, chopped

½ onion, chopped

1 bay leaf

3 cups beef bone broth

1 teaspoon fresh thyme

¼ teaspoon dried sage

¼ teaspoon black pepper + additional to taste

1 cup whole milk

½ cup cream

4 large heads black garlic, flesh squeezed out of paper husks (can substitute roasted regular garlic)

Coconut oil or tallow for frying

Handful fresh sage leaves, parsley, or oregano

Flaked sea salt

1. Preheat the oven to 425°F. Place the marrowbones on a baking sheet lined with foil and drizzle them with 1 tablespoon olive oil and ½ teaspoon sea salt. Place the bones in the oven and roast for 20–25 minutes. Remove the bones from the oven and set them aside to cool.

2. Melt the butter in a large saucepan over medium-low heat. Add the shallots, onion, and bay leaf and cook until the onions have softened and are translucent, about 20 minutes. While the onions and shallots are cooking, scoop the jellied marrow out of the bones and set aside. Reserve the bones.

3. Once the onions have cooked sufficiently, add the broth, thyme, sage, black pepper, and bones. Bring the heat down to low and simmer, uncovered, for 30 minutes, stirring every 15 minutes. Add the milk, cream, marrowbones, and garlic. Remove the bones from the soup with a slotted spoon.

4. Blend the soup mixture in batches in a high-powered blender or food processor until velvety smooth. Pour the soup back into the pot, bring to a simmer over low heat, and salt to taste. Remove from the heat and set aside, covered, while preparing the garnish.

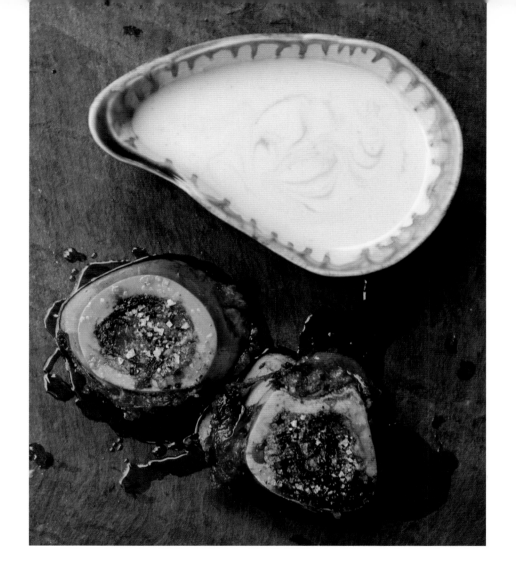

5. To prepare the crispy herbs, heat a few tablespoons coconut oil or tallow in a small skillet until hot. Add the herbs and fry until crispy, just a few seconds for herbs with thin leaves. Remove the herbs and place them on a plate lined with paper towels. Immediately sprinkle the leaves with flaked sea salt.

6. Distribute the soup into serving bowls and top with crispy herbs and a grind of black pepper. Serve immediately.

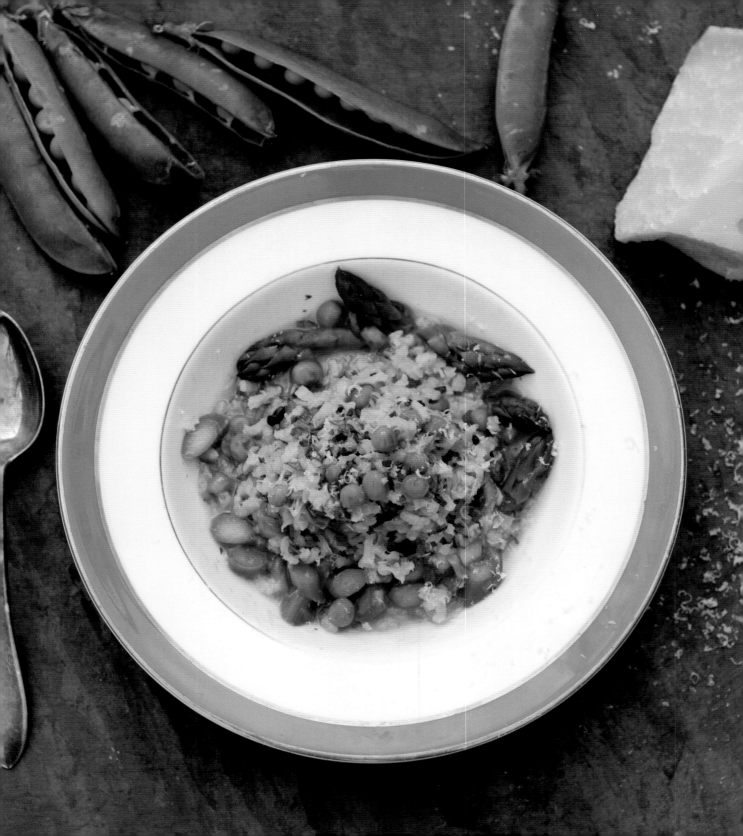

Risotto with Asparagus, Sweet Peas, and Tarragon

OF THE TRADITIONAL RECIPES THAT MAKE USE OF LARGER AMOUNTS OF BROTH AT ONCE, RISOTTO IS an obvious choice. The shape of the rice grain used for making risottos, such as arborio and carnaroli, is stubby, sticky, and fast-cooking. Using bone broth as the cooking liquid for risotto imparts so much flavor and creaminess to this dish. Substitute the vegetables for what's local and seasonal in your area.

Yield: 4–6 servings

⅔ cup fresh shelled or frozen peas

8 medium asparagus spears, chopped

5–6 cups beef bone broth

1 tablespoon butter, divided use

2 tablespoons olive oil, divided use

1 small onion, chopped

4 thyme sprigs, leaves picked and stems discarded

1 cup carnaroli rice (can substitute arborio, but the consistency will be softer and stickier)

2 cloves garlic, minced

1 cup white wine (you may omit and use more broth instead)

1 tablespoon capers

¼ cup grated Parmesan cheese (raw sheep's milk Parmesan is delicious if you can find it)

Salt and pepper to taste

1 handful chopped fresh tarragon (substitute parsley, basil, or mint)

1. Fill a medium pot with water and bring to a boil. Have a mixing bowl ready with ice water. Add a small handful of salt to the pot and bring the water back to a boil. Add the peas and blanch for 30 seconds or until barely cooked and still firm. Use a spider skimmer or a slotted spoon to remove and shock the peas in the ice water. Drain the peas in a colander and set aside. Use the same pot to blanch the asparagus in the same way.

2. In a small pot, warm up the bone broth and keep it warm nearby.

3. In a large heavy-bottomed pot, warm up 1½ teaspoons olive oil and 1 tablespoon butter over medium heat and sauté the onions with thyme. When the onions become soft, add the remaining olive oil and butter. Add the rice and garlic. Mix well to coat the rice evenly with the butter and oil, and stir until the rice turns golden and fragrant, 2–3 minutes. Add the wine and stir continuously until the wine has completely evaporated. Ladle in the bone broth, ½ cup at a time, stirring all along. Wait until each addition of broth has been absorbed before adding more.

4. When the risotto is thoroughly cooked, add the capers and lightly stir to coat evenly. Immediately add the blanched peas and asparagus. Turn off the heat and add the Parmesan, lightly stirring one last time. Season with salt and pepper to taste. Serve with freshly chopped tarragon.

Lentils Braised in Beef Bone Broth with Leeks, Tomato, Butternut Squash, and Plantain

THIS STEW IS INSPIRED BY A FAVORITE SOUP SERVED AT A RESTAURANT LYA'S DAD USED TO take her to on the weekends—a warming bowl of steaming hot lentils in tomato broth with chunks of fried plantain. This version is more of a stew, with a lot more body and heartiness, to be served as a single-dish meal or as an entree. It's especially lovely in the fall.

Yield: 4–6 servings

1½ cups French lentils

Filtered water

1 tablespoon lemon juice or apple cider vinegar

3 tomatoes

2 tablespoons coconut oil, divided use

1 large leek, chopped

1 teaspoon dried thyme

1 teaspoon dried oregano

¼ teaspoon fresh ground pepper

½ teaspoon cumin seeds

2 cups butternut squash, diced (1 inch dice)

1 quart beef bone broth

1 teaspoon sea salt + additional to taste

1 green plantain, diced or sliced (optional)

GARNISH

Cilantro or parsley, chopped

1. Soak the lentils overnight in 3 cups water with lemon juice or apple cider vinegar to neutralize phytic acid (phytic acid binds important nutrients and can hinder their absorption). Drain and rinse.

2. Fill a small pot with water and bring to a boil. Have a mixing bowl ready with ice water. Add the tomatoes to the boiling water. When their skins break, remove them from the pot and place them in the ice water. Peel and chop the tomatoes.

3. Sauté the leeks in 1 tablespoon coconut oil in a large, heavy-bottomed pot. Add the thyme, oregano, pepper, and cumin. When the leeks soften, add the tomatoes and butternut squash.

4. When the squash softens, add the lentils and mix well with the rest of the ingredients in the pot. Add the beef bone broth and sea salt. Bring to a boil, turn down the heat, and simmer for about 1 hour or until the lentils are fully cooked. Season with more salt to taste. If you like a more soupy consistency, add more water and simmer a little longer.

5. While the lentils are simmering, warm the remaining 1 tablespoon coconut oil in a frying pan. Add the diced or sliced plantain and brown on all sides.

6. Serve the lentils with sautéed plantains and a sprinkle of chopped cilantro or parsley.

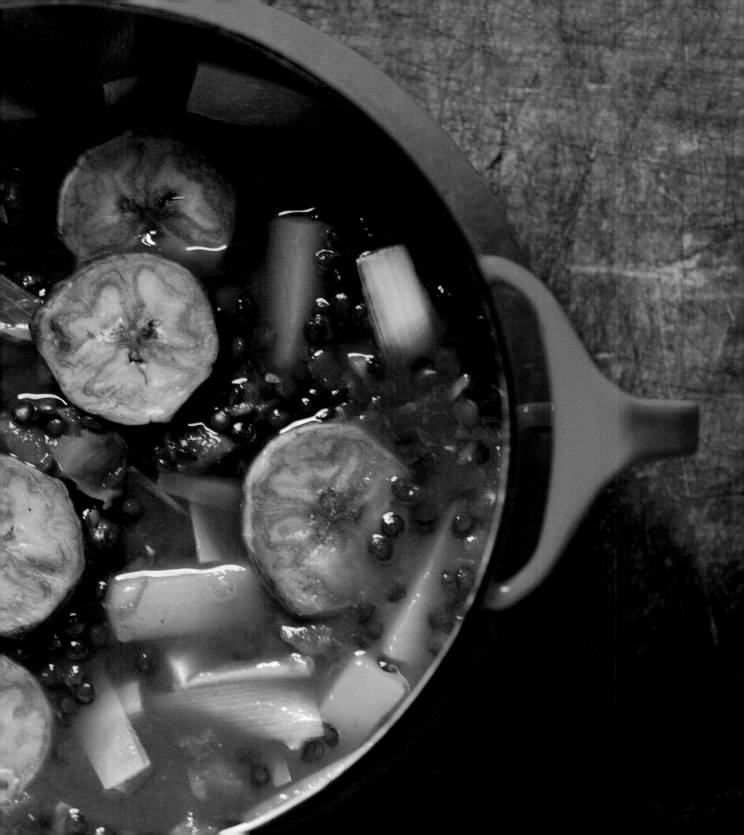

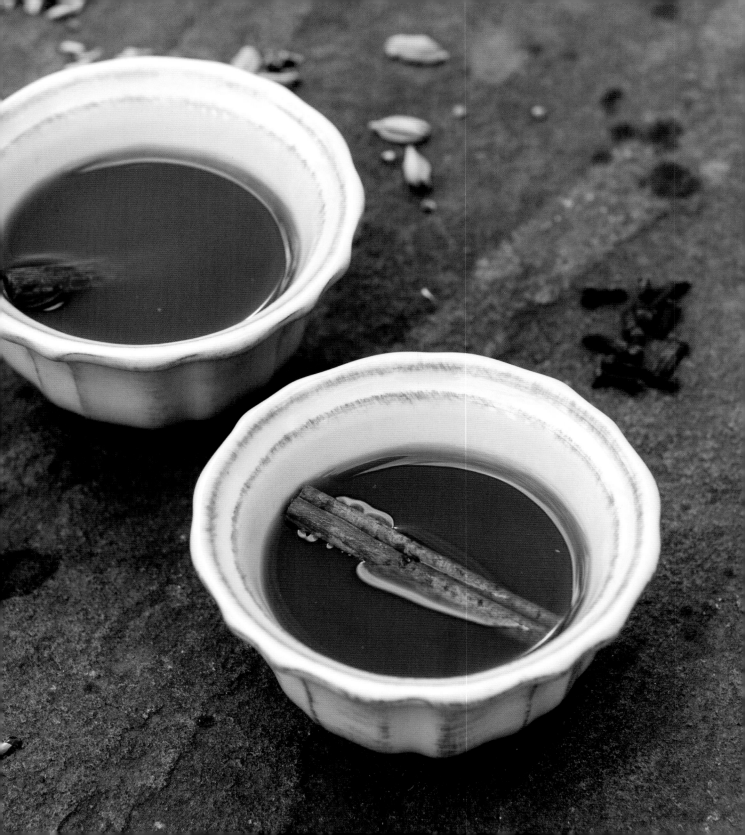

Bone Broth Warming Tea

THIS TEA IS AN EXAMPLE OF A RECIPE WHERE THE FLAVOR OF BONE BROTH IS DIFFICULT to trace. The root and spice combination is strong and naturally sweet, masking the broth's flavor. This blend has a warming and stimulating effect in the body, and complements bone broth's digestive enhancing properties. For a less stimulating effect, omit the black tea leaves. If you don't like the sweet taste of licorice, you could add honey or maple syrup to your taste.

Yield: 2 servings

1 cup beef bone broth

½ cup water

1 teaspoon licorice root chips (or 1 licorice tea bag)

2 cardamom pods

1 cinnamon stick (2½ inches long)

½ teaspoon black peppercorns

1 tablespoon loose black tea leaves (or 1 black tea bag)

Milk, for serving (optional)

1. In a small saucepan, bring the bone broth, water, licorice, cardamom, cinnamon, and peppercorns to a boil. Reduce the heat to low, cover the pot, and simmer for 15 minutes.

2. Add the black tea, turn off the heat, and let it steep for 5 minutes.

3. Strain the tea and serve with milk or dilute it with a little water. Serve warm or cold.

A NOTE ON DAIRY

Our stance on dairy is quality or none at all. This rings true for both real dairy and alternative milks. When purchasing animal dairy, always look for grass-fed, unhomogenized, whole, and, if available, raw products. Grass-fed dairy contains more omega-3s and vitamin E. Raw milk is preferable, especially for those with lactose sensitivity, because the enzymes needed to absorb the nutrients in milk are still present. Lipase, which is necessary for digesting fats; lactase, which allows us to digest lactose; and phosphatase, which helps us process calcium, are all present in unpasteurized milk.

Whole milk contains the appropriate amount of fat (nature's perfect design at it again) to carry vitamins A and D, which are necessary for the absorption of calcium.

When using nut or grain milks, avoid store-bought, with the exception of unsweetened, full-fat coconut milk. Boxed alternative milks too often contain unnecessary fillers and preservatives, and they are not easily tolerated because they are generally made without properly sprouting the nuts, seeds, or grains (sprouting reduces the phytic acid content and enhances digestibility).

Sunday Five-Hour Bolognese

THIS BOLOGNESE IS MAGICAL. WE CAN'T HELP BUT GET EXCITED SPENDING A SUNDAY afternoon watching the broth simmer into this sauce, patiently waiting to polish it off with the final cup of fresh milk, and pat of cultured butter, before sharing with our friends and family. Even the aroma that fills the apartment makes it feel decidedly more home-y.

This bolognese truly can stand alone as the main event. It's served more like a chili, and perfect with a bright green salad dressed with your best olive oil and a hunk of crunchy, chewy sourdough.

Yield: 6 servings

3 tablespoons extra virgin olive oil

2 medium carrots, peeled and finely chopped

2 stalks celery, finely chopped

2 medium onions, finely chopped

½ pound pancetta, finely chopped (substitute with prosciutto if necessary)

1½ pounds lean ground beef

½ pound ground pork butt (you can use all ground beef if pork is unavailable)

1 tablespoon tomato paste

8 cups beef broth, divided use

2½ cups whole milk (grass-fed is best)

5 tablespoons butter

Kosher salt and ground black pepper

1. In a large, deep sauté pan, heat the olive oil over high heat. Add the carrots, celery, and onions. Cook, stirring until the vegetables are lightly browned, for about 6 minutes. Add the pancetta and cook, stirring, for 2 minutes. Add the beef and cook another 2 minutes. Add pork and cook until the meat is lightly browned, about 5 minutes.

2. Whisk together the tomato paste and 1 cup broth, and add it to the meat mixture. Reduce the heat to low so that sauce just barely simmers. When the broth has evaporated, add another cup. Continue to cook, stirring occasionally and adding a cup of broth when stew becomes dry, until all the broth has been added, about 4 hours.

3. Add the milk and butter, and continue to simmer very gently until the milk is evaporated and the sauce is very thick, about 1¼ hours. Season to taste with salt and pepper, and serve as desired.

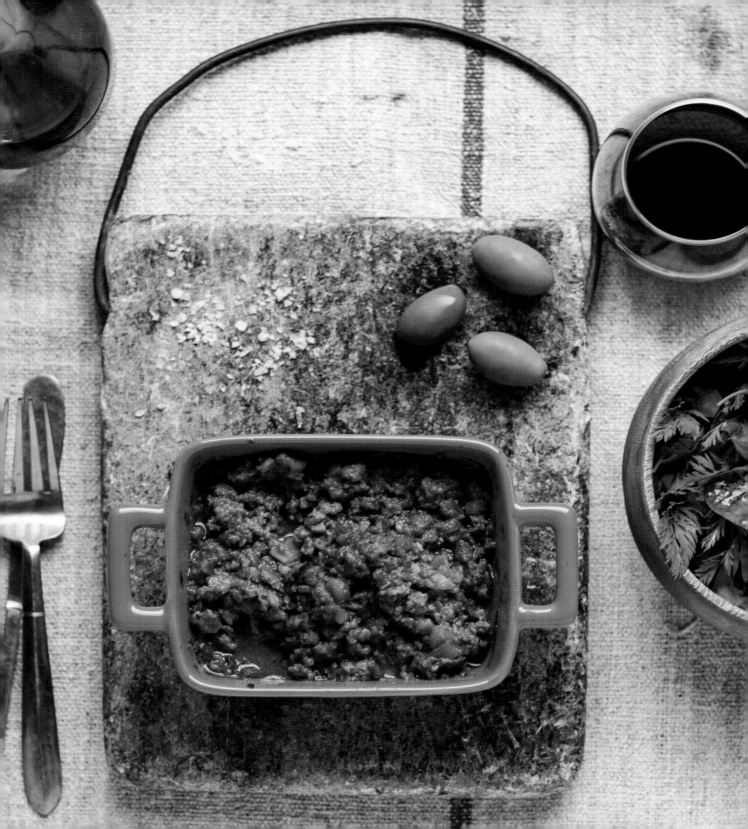

Spanish Squid over Borlotti Beans

THIS RECIPE IS INSPIRED BY TAYLOR'S ALL-TIME FAVORITE DISH SERVED AT APRIL BLOOMFIELD'S
restaurant The John Dory: the chorizo-stuffed squid. With tart sherry vinegar, savory chorizo,
creamy borlotti beans, and decadent crème fraîche, there's an incredible fusion of flavors here.
Baby squid are remarkably easy to work with, and each layer of the composed dish
can be prepared in advance, in bulk, and used in other recipes.

Yield: 4 servings

1 tablespoon + 2 teaspoons olive oil + additional for roasting the squid, divided use

½ cup crushed tomatoes, rinsed and strained

1 tablespoon sherry vinegar

½ teaspoon coconut sugar

¼ cup ground chorizo (optional)

½ yellow onion, minced

½ red bell pepper, minced

1 pinch saffron

¼ teaspoon paprika

Salt and pepper to taste

½ cup presoaked white rice (any short grain white paella or risotto rice will work)

4 cups beef bone broth

2 cups presoaked borlotti beans

8 baby squid bodies + 4 tentacles (baby squid can sometimes be difficult to find, in which case you can use just 10 tentacles)

2 tablespoons crème fraîche

Fresh cilantro

1. In a small saucepan, warm 1 tablespoon olive oil over medium-high heat. Add the tomatoes, sherry vinegar, and sugar and cook, stirring regularly, until the liquid reduces, roughly 5 minutes. Remove from the heat and set aside.

2. Add 1 teaspoon of the remaining olive oil to the pan and add the chorizo. Cook for 2 minutes, then add the onion and bell pepper. Cook until the vegetables are softened. Add the saffron, paprika, and salt to taste and continue cooking until the onion begins to caramelize.

3. In a rice cooker or heavy-bottomed saucepot, add the rice, 1 cup broth, the remaining 1 teaspoon olive oil, and the chorizo mixture. Cover and cook until the liquid is gone, about 20 minutes.

4. In a separate small saucepot, bring the remaining 3 cups broth to a boil and add the beans. Cook until the flesh of the beans is creamy and a little broth remains, roughly 30 minutes.

5. Coat the squid with olive oil, salt, and pepper. If you are able to find baby squid bodies, stuff them with the rice mixture before broiling. Broil the squid until it just begins to char.

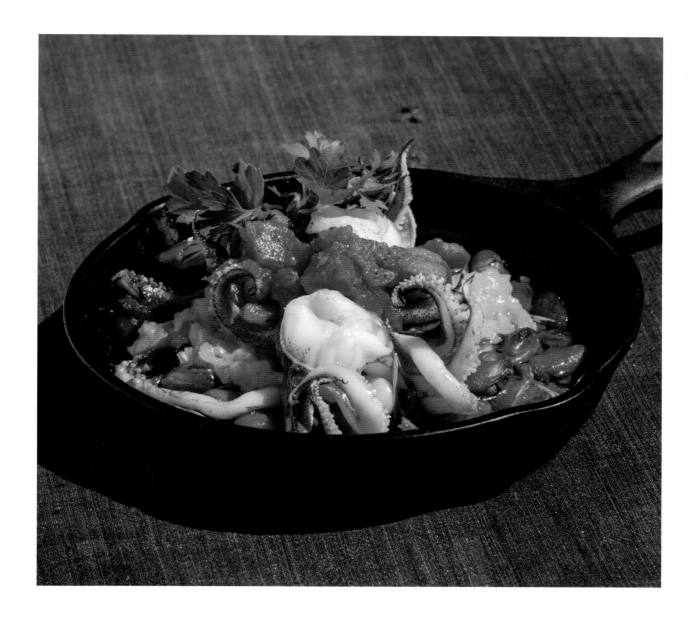

6. In a small cast-iron pan or four oven-safe wide ramekins, spoon the beans to layer the bottom, add a dollop of crème fraîche, and stir to melt. Over the bean layer, spoon some of the chorizo-rice mixture and top with the squid. Atop the squid, spoon the tomato mixture. Garnish with fresh cilantro.

BEEF OR BISON

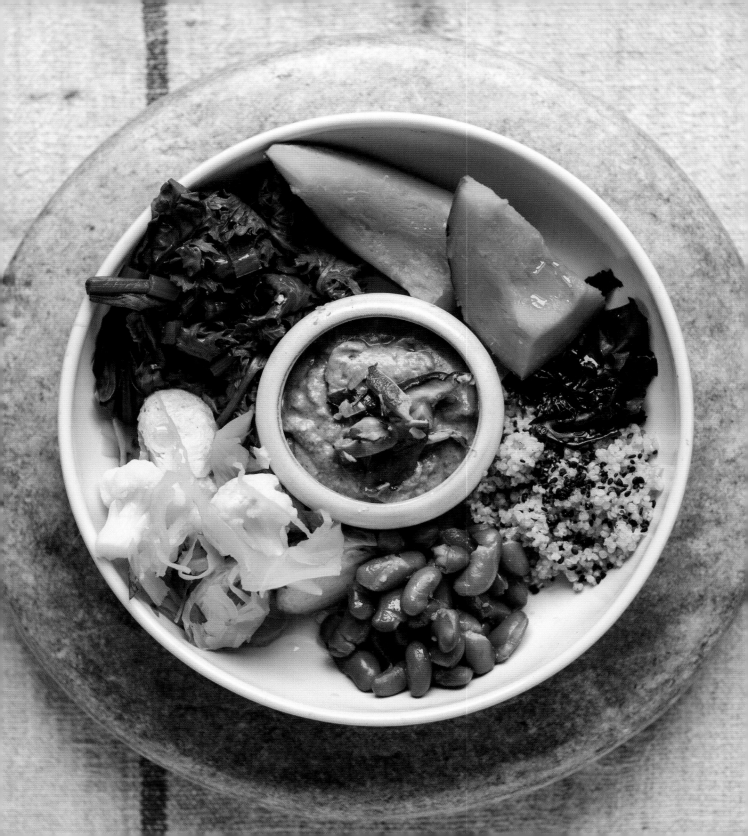

The Macro Bowl, Reinvented

THIS NONTRADITIONAL MACRO BOWL HIGHLIGHTS BONE BROTH IN THE SAUCE: a shiitake mushroom gravy. The added bone broth facilitates digestion of all the other foods, enhancing the health benefits of this bowl. Shiitake mushrooms are commonly used in Chinese medicine to support the healthy flow of energy in the body, and to tonify the blood. This shiitake mushroom gravy has a deep earthy and umami flavor. At home, we also love it over roasted vegetables, on steak, or with roast chicken. When refrigerated, it becomes very thick, and if brought to room temperature it can be served as a dip for crudités, bread, chips, and crackers.

Yield: About 2½ cups

1 tablespoon olive oil

1 tablespoon butter

1½ cups onion, chopped (1 medium)

4–5 sprigs thyme, leaves picked and chopped

2–3 sprigs rosemary, leaves picked and chopped

1 pound shiitake mushrooms, stems removed, sliced (save the stems to add to your next pot of bone broth)

4 cloves garlic, minced

2 cups beef bone broth

1 teaspoon salt or nama shoyu (soy sauce)

1.   Heat the olive oil in a skillet. Add the butter and sauté the onions over medium heat with the thyme and rosemary. When the onions soften, add the mushrooms. When the mushrooms have released their moisture and wilted, about 10–15 minutes, add the garlic. Cook for another 3 minutes, then add the bone broth. Bring to a boil, reduce the heat, and simmer for about 15–20 minutes.

2.   Transfer to a blender, leaving a few sautéed mushrooms behind for garnish. Blend until smooth. If the gravy is too thick, loosen it a little by placing it in a saucepot over low-medium heat, and adding a little more broth to your desired consistency.

3.   Add salt or shoyu and serve.

MAKING A MACRO BOWL

Lya's favorite macro bowl includes steamed quinoa, pinto beans, lightly sautéed seasonal vegetables, a chunk of baked winter squash or sweet potato, dulse seaweed, and bone broth–braised greens, with a little lacto-fermented cabbage as garnish. Experiment with your favorite choice of grains, beans, seaweed, and vegetables. Adding fermented vegetables provides an extra healthful boost, as they contain probiotics—the friendly bacteria that we need for healthy microflora in our guts.

Bone Broth–Braised Red Cabbage with Bacon and Apples

ONCE UPON A TIME, IN A FAR AWAY LAND, TAYLOR WAS VEGETARIAN. (SHHH, DON'T TELL!) Her husband, Chris, loves to tell the story of how he converted Taylor back to the other side. Still, there are days when just veggies feels good. This braised cabbage is inspired by a similar dish Taylor loved in her vegetarian days. This recipe shines in autumn when the apples are in peak season and cabbages are coming around. Though bacon is included in this variation, it is optional, of course.

Yield: 6–8 servings as a side dish

4 ounces bacon (about 4 slices), cut crosswise into ½ inch pieces

1 medium red onion, thinly sliced

1 apple, cored and diced (we used local Macintosh, but you might try Golden Delicious, Macoun, or any other sweet and crunchy variety)

1 small or ½ large head red cabbage, halved, cored, and cut lengthwise into ¼ inch thick slices

¼ cup cider vinegar

1½ cups beef broth

1 tablespoon maple syrup

1½ teaspoons salt

1. Add bacon to a skillet over medium heat and cook, stirring occasionally, until crisp. Remove the bacon and drain the excess fat from the pan, leaving just a light coating.

2. Add the onion and apples to the pan and cook, stirring occasionally, until the onion is translucent and the apples soften. Add the cabbage, vinegar, broth, maple syrup, and salt; stir to combine. Raise the heat to medium-high, cover, and cook for 5 minutes.

3. Return the bacon to the cabbage mixture and reduce the heat to medium-low. Continue to cook, covered, stirring occasionally, 30 to 60 minutes. We usually give it an hour for the cabbage to soften and the subtle sweetness to come through the reduced broth.

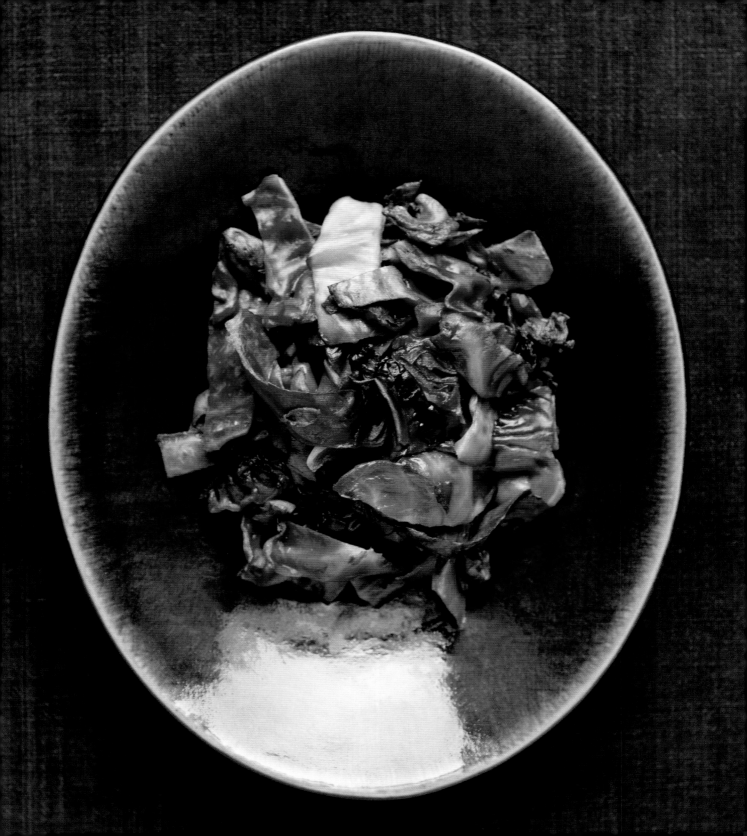

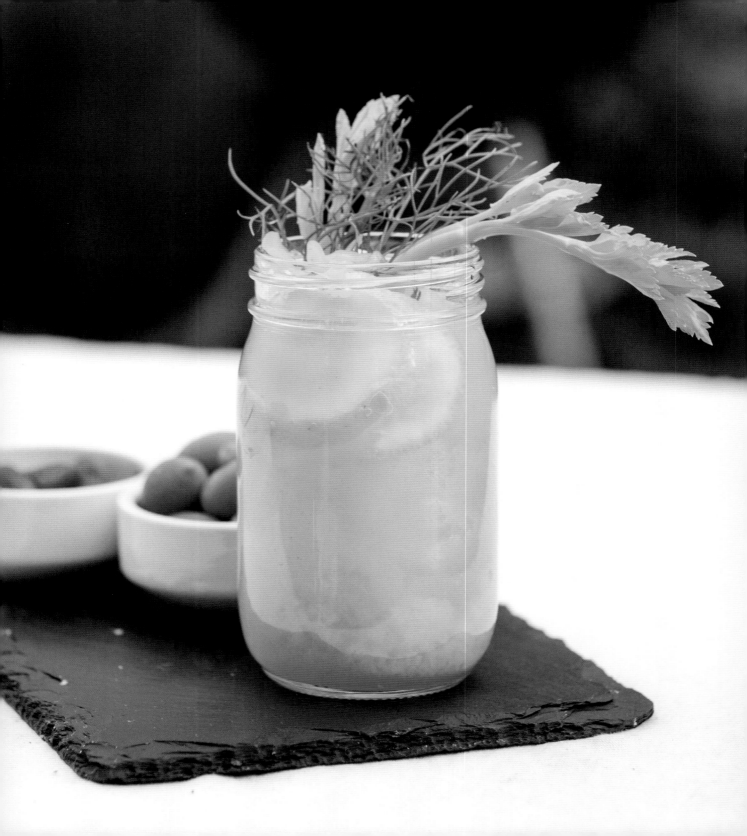

Bone Broth Bloody Mary, aka the Bullshot

THIS LONG-LOST CLASSIC COCKTAIL TRACES BACK TO THE 1950S, WHEN A *BROADWAY* JOURNALIST
predicted the drink would catch on like wildfire "because it's so full of vitamins!"
The boozy, brothy beverage indeed caught on and quickly won over the Hollywood crowd.
Richard Chamberlain and Joan Crawford were said to have gotten drunk on Bullshots
lunching at La Grenouille in New York City, and even decades later, the drink was Malcolm
McDowell's go-to order on his press tour for *A Clockwork Orange.*

When researching the history of the Bullshot, we were instantly tickled by how closely
it's paralleled the broth resurgence as of late. Rumor has it the drink is still available today
at a few old-school New York City steak houses and theater district haunts, if you know who to ask.
But, I foresee the Bullshot renaissance coming soon!

Yield: 1 serving

1½ ounces vodka

2½ ounces beef broth

Juice of 1 lemon wedge

2 dashes Worcestershire sauce

2 dashes Tabasco sauce

Freshly ground black pepper

Shake the vodka, broth, lemon juice, Worcestershire sauce, and Tabasco sauce well with ice, then strain into an old-fashioned glass full of fresh ice. Garnish with a full twist of fresh black pepper.

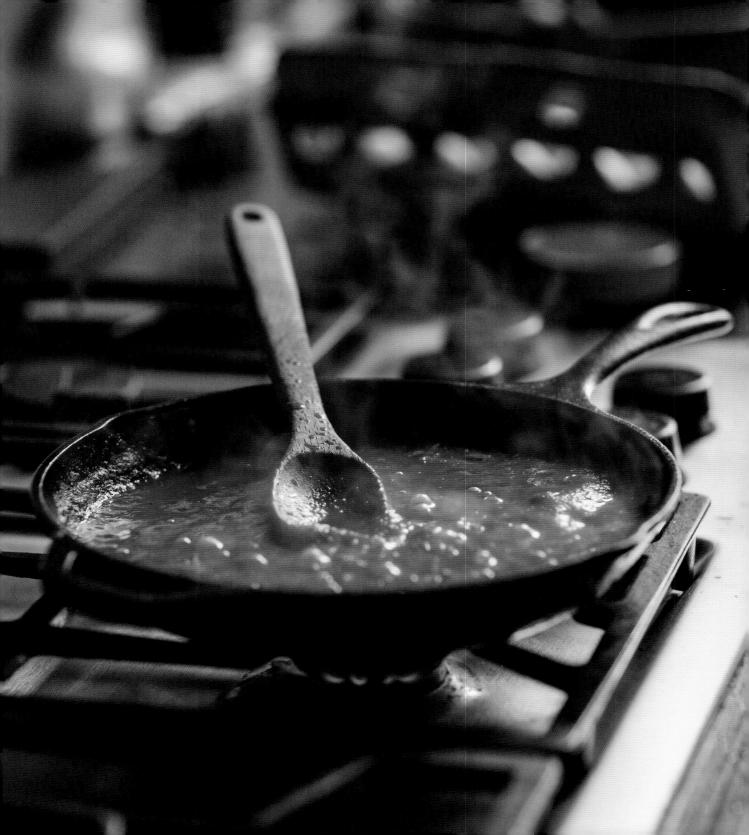

"There are marked improvements in my blood sugar levels when I drink lots of bone broth. Additionally, I noticed that once I started drinking bone broth, my cravings for almost every food went away. One might still say that yes, I want a cookie, but do I have that visceral craving for one anymore? No, not since starting to drink the broth."

—*Keith Curbow,*
JAZZ MUSICIAN WHO HAS LIVED WITH
TYPE 1 DIABETES AND HAS KEPT HIMSELF
OFF INSULIN SINCE 2013 USING DIET, MOVEMENT,
AND MEDITATION TO BECOME INSULIN-INDEPENDENT

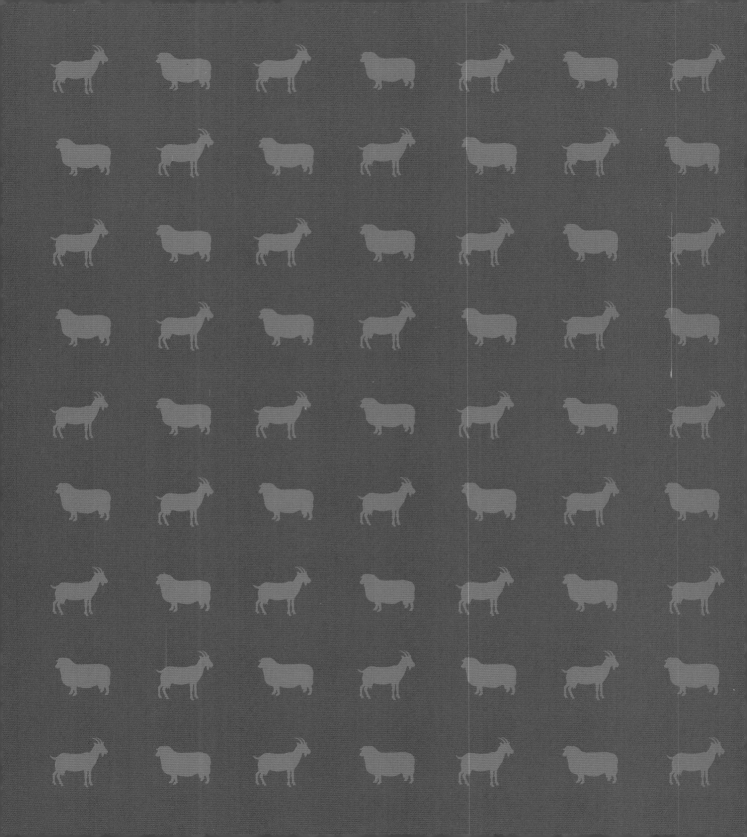

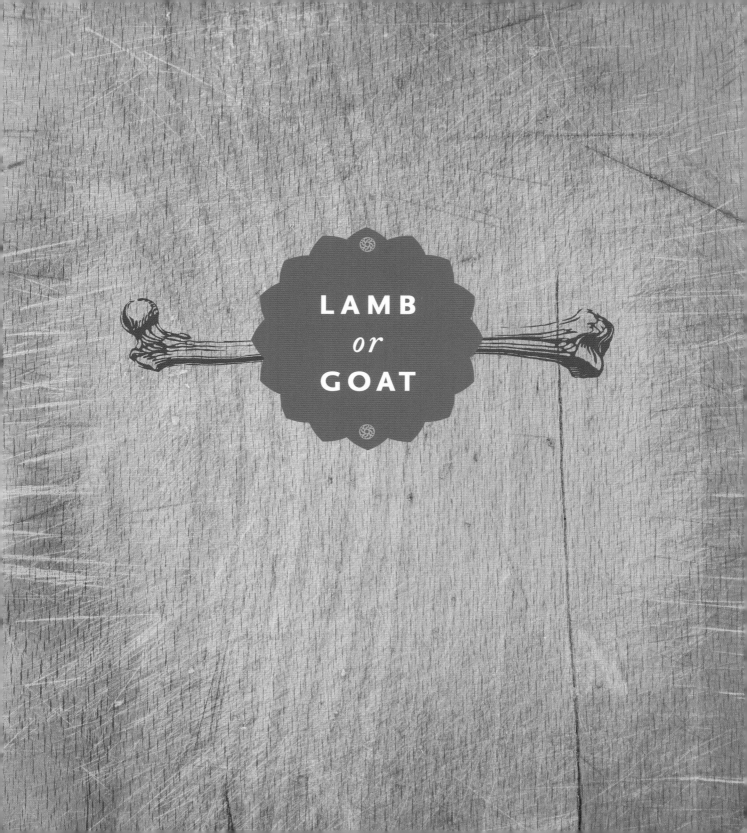

LAMB

or

GOAT

Swiss Chard Rolls Filled with Braised Oxtails and Red Wine Sauce

OXTAIL MEAT IS DECADENT WHEN SLOW COOKED FOR HOURS. IT MELTS OFF THE BONE, making it a great choice for stews. For this recipe you will need to plan ahead of time: one night to marinate, the next day to slowly cook the meat, and another day to allow for the flavors to merge. The wait will pay off! Wrapping the meat in swiss chard leaves makes for a gorgeous presentation and a different way of enjoying a classic stew.

Yield: 6 servings

5 pounds oxtails

3 carrots, chopped

4 celery stalks, chopped

1 onion, roughly chopped

A few sprigs fresh herbs, such as thyme, rosemary, bay leaves, or oregano

6 cloves garlic, smashed

1 tablespoon allspice or juniper berries

2 tablespoons peppercorns

Peel of 1 orange, slivered

4 cups red wine

⅓ cup plus 2 tablespoons olive oil, divided use

6 cups beef or lamb bone broth

Salt

12 Swiss chard leaves

1. In a large bowl, place the oxtails, carrots, celery, onion, herbs, garlic, allspice, peppercorns, orange peel, wine, and ⅓ cup olive oil. Cover and marinate overnight.

2. Remove the meat from the marinade and set the marinade aside. Heat the remaining 2 tablespoons olive oil over medium heat and brown the oxtails on all sides. Transfer the browned oxtails to a plate. Place the oxtails in a Dutch oven or a large, heavy-bottomed pot and pour the marinating juices and vegetables over the meat. Add the bone broth and bring to a boil. Reduce the heat and simmer for 2–4 hours. The longer you cook it over low heat, the softer the meat will get.

3. Turn off the heat and let the oxtails cool. Using tongs, remove the meat and set it aside. Strain the cooking sauce and discard the vegetables and aromatics. When the meat is cool enough to handle, pick it from the bones and discard the bones. Pour the strained sauce over the meat and refrigerate.

4. The next day, remove the oxtails and sauce from the refrigerator and skim off some of the fat that has congealed on top of the sauce. Warm the meat with its sauce over medium-low heat. Strain the meat from the sauce, transfer it to a bowl, and cover. Bring the sauce to a boil, reduce the heat a little, and leave it to simmer until the sauce reduces by half.

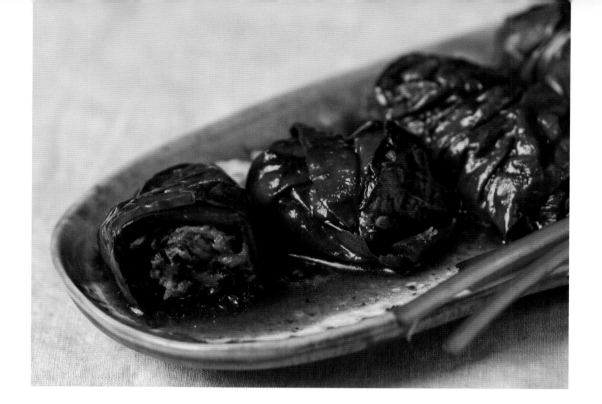

5. Bring a large pot of water to a boil. Prepare a large bowl with ice water and have it ready near the stove. Remove the extra stems from the chard so that you are left with the leaf only. When the water is boiling, add a small handful of salt to the water and stir. Add the chard leaves to the boiling water and blanch them for 15–20 seconds. Remove them from the pot using tongs or a spider skimmer. Transfer to the ice water, and then pat them dry with a kitchen cloth.

6. Place the chard so that the center stem is aligned vertically in front of you. Put 2–3 spoonfuls of the warm meat in the middle, depending on the size of the leaves. Using your hands, fold the top and bottom edges of the leaf over the meat. Then, starting from the left edge of the leaf, begin to roll the leaf toward the right edge of the leaf, similarly to making burritos. Spoon half of the reduced sauce in the middle of a serving plate and place the rolls over it. Spoon the remaining sauce on top of the rolls and serve immediately. Enjoy with a side of roasted vegetables, mashed potatoes, sweet potatoes, or your grain of choice.

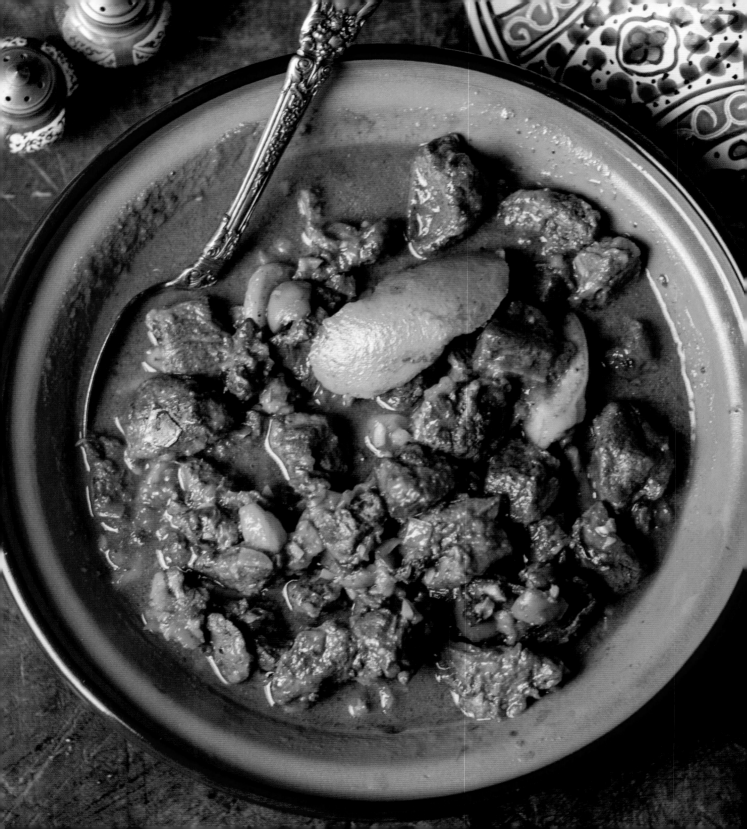

Lamb Tagine with Apricot, Green Olive, and Preserved Lemon

THIS DISH, THOUGH LAYERED AND COMPLEX, IS QUITE SIMPLE TO PREPARE.
We use this basic recipe year-round and enjoy substituting quartered chicken thighs or vegetables in place of the lamb during warmer months. If using vegetables, our favorites include summer or winter squashes, onions, and fennel. We recommend investing in a proper tagine dish for cooking; it truly elevates the experience and makes for a stunning presentation!

Yield: 4–6 servings

1 cinnamon stick

1 teaspoon whole black pepper-corns

1 teaspoon cumin seeds

1 teaspoon sweet or hot paprika

1 teaspoon red pepper flakes

¼ teaspoon whole cloves

5 tablespoons extra virgin olive oil, divided use

4 cloves garlic, sliced

1 teaspoon chopped fresh ginger root

1 handful fresh cilantro leaves, chopped

2 bay leaves

1 large pinch saffron

2–3 cups cubed lamb meat

Kosher salt

Freshly ground black pepper

1 medium onion, coarsely chopped

1 preserved lemon (recipe p. 78)

½ cup cracked green olives

⅓ cup dried apricots

1 cup lamb or chicken bone broth

1. In a skillet over medium heat, toast the cinnamon, peppercorns, cumin, paprika, red pepper flakes, and cloves until they start to smoke. Remove from the heat and grind in a spice grinder.

2. In a bowl large enough to accommodate the lamb, combine 3 tablespoons olive oil with the spice mix, garlic, ginger, cilantro, bay leaves, and saffron. Mix to form a paste. Add the lamb, rubbing the marinade over all the pieces. Cover and refrigerate for 2 hours or overnight.

3. In a tagine or large casserole dish over medium-high heat, heat the remaining 2 tablespoons olive oil. Add the lamb pieces and lightly brown on all sides, about 5 minutes. Add the onion and cook until it just starts to brown, about 3 minutes.

4. Rinse the preserved lemon well. Scoop out the flesh and discard. Cut the peel into strips and add to the pan. Add the olives, apricots, and broth. Cover tightly and cook over medium-low heat for 30–35 minutes.

5. Remove the bay leaves and discard. Serve warm over long-grain rice or on its own.

(Continued)

1. Boil 4 cleaned lemons (we especially like Meyer lemons if available) until soft (10 minutes).

2. Transfer lemons to ice water and reserve cooking liquid.

3. Score lemons as if cutting in quarters, but leave them intact.

4. Whisk together ⅓ cup sugar, 6 tablespoons salt, 1 teaspoon coriander seeds, 1 clove, and 3 cups of the warm cooking liquid.

5. Transfer lemons to a glass Mason jar and add brine to cover completely.

6. Seal and chill at least 2 weeks.

ORGAN MEATS

Many traditional cultures, and even the pre-drug medical profession, believed that eating the organs from a healthy animal would support the organs of the eater. Often, the traditional way to treat a person with an organ weakness or imbalance was to feed them the same organ from a healthy animal. Even in modern times, a number of people who need thyroid hormones have eaten the thyroid glands of animals and reported this as an effective alternative to thyroid medication. While we do not suggest self-prescribing organ meats as medicine, we do know, and research has proven, that organ meats are storehouses for super nutrition.

While few people love the taste of organ meats, we found ourselves craving liver during our pregnancies and still while nursing. Most people need a little persuading. Ground meat dishes, like our bolognese (p. 60), are an easy place to sneak in nutrient-dense organ meats. Offal in the form of heart, liver, kidneys, and tongue are chock full of nutrition, and just a small amount supplies tremendous nutritional value. Heart meat is the best source of CoQ10—great for heart health and helping us deal with oxidative stress—that you can find. Liver supplies incredible amounts of vitamin A, vitamin B12, choline, and folate. Kidneys provide a jolt of protein and amino acids. Tongue meat is rich in iron, B vitamins, choline, zinc, and trace minerals.

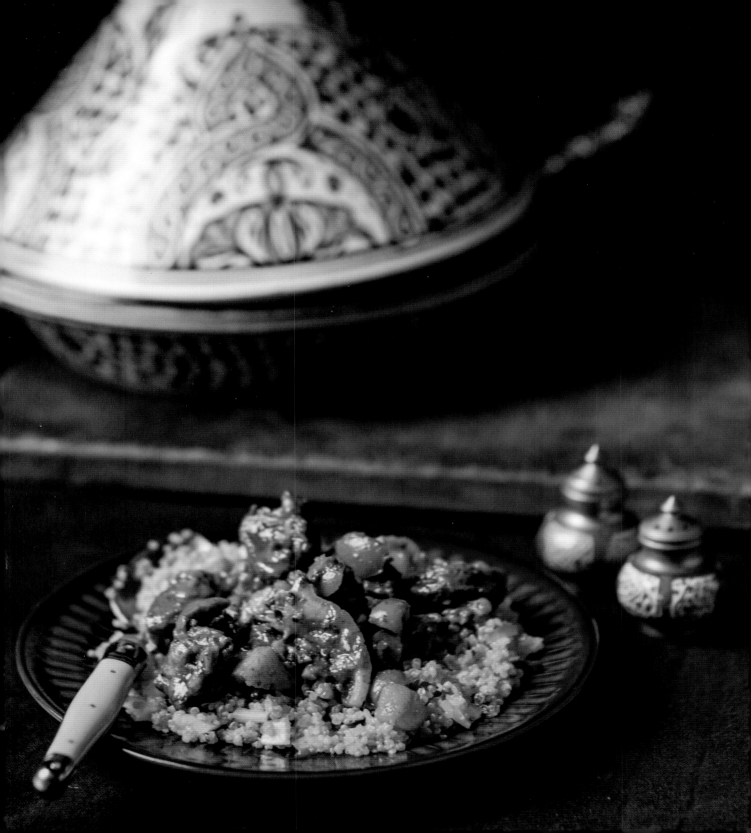

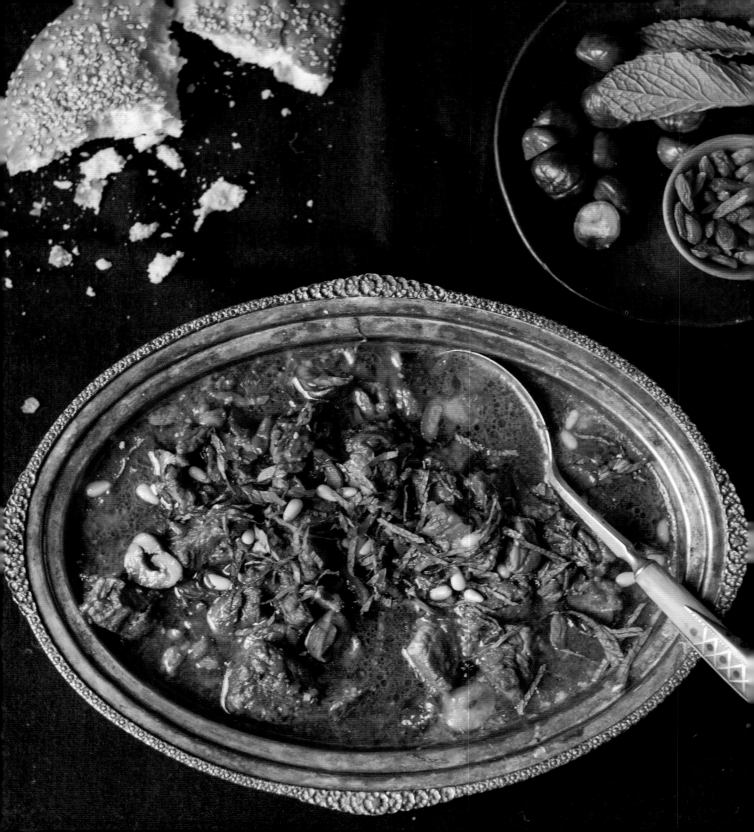

Lamb Stew with Chestnuts, Honey, Saffron, and Goji Berries

LAMB IS CONSIDERED THE MOST HEAT-INDUCING MEAT IN CHINESE MEDICINE, PERFECT FOR cold winter nights. Substitute goji berries with dates, apricots, or fresh pomegranate seeds. If you use dates or apricots, add them during the last 30 minutes of cooking. If you use goji berries or pomegranate seeds, be sure to add them at the very end to retain their vibrant rose color.

Yield: 6 servings

2 tablespoons coconut oil or ghee

2 onions, chopped

4 garlic cloves, minced

1 inch piece ginger root, peeled and chopped

1 pinch saffron

2 cinnamon sticks (each about 2 inches long)

3 pounds boneless shoulder of lamb, cubed

4 cups lamb or beef bone broth

1 cup peeled and roasted chestnuts

2 tablespoons honey (preferably a dark honey)

Salt and pepper to taste

⅓ cup goji berries

GARNISH

Chopped cilantro

1. In a heavy-bottomed pot, warm the coconut oil or ghee and sauté the onions. When they begin to soften, add the garlic and ginger root. Mix thoroughly. After a couple of minutes, add the saffron and cinnamon sticks. Add the lamb and brown on all sides.

2. Pour the bone broth in the pot until it barely covers the lamb. Turn the heat up and bring to a boil. Reduce the heat, cover, and simmer for 1–2 hours or until the lamb becomes very tender.

3. Add the chestnuts and honey and simmer for 30 more minutes. Season to taste with salt and pepper. Sprinkle the goji berries over the stew, turn off the heat, and let it rest for a few minutes.

4. Serve immediately or let it rest overnight and serve the day after—the flavors will merge, making the stew even more delicious. Garnish with chopped cilantro just before serving.

Quinoa and Artichoke Salad
with Lemon, Capers, Parsley, and Thyme

QUINOA, THE ANCIENT ANDEAN STAPLE, HAS IN RECENT YEARS REACHED SUPERFOOD STATUS. In comparison to other grains (quinoa is not actually a grain, but rather a pseudo-cereal), quinoa is gluten-free and comparatively high in protein. Quinoa boasts a favorable amino acid profile, with generous lysine content in particular. It is also a good source of B vitamins, iron, magnesium, and phosphorous. Cooking sprouted quinoa with broth, and serving with just vegetables keeps it easy on the belly.

Yield: 4 servings

2–3 tablespoons olive oil, divided use

1 cup sweet or yellow onion, chopped

½ teaspoon chopped fresh thyme

1 (9-ounce) package frozen artichoke hearts, thawed

1 cup lamb bone broth

½ cup uncooked, soaked, and sprouted quinoa (you can find already sprouted quinoa in some health food stores—it is a great time saver!)

1 cup chopped fresh parsley

3 teaspoons grated lemon zest

1½ tablespoons fresh lemon juice

¼ teaspoon kosher salt

1. Heat 1 tablespoon olive oil in a medium saucepan over medium-high heat. Add the onion and thyme and sauté 5 minutes or until onion is tender.

2. Add the artichokes and sauté 2 minutes or until thoroughly heated. Add the broth and quinoa and bring to a simmer. Cover and cook 18 minutes or until the liquid is completely absorbed.

3. Remove the pan from the heat. Stir in the parsley, lemon zest, lemon juice, salt, and the remaining 1–2 tablespoons olive oil. Serve warm or at room temperature.

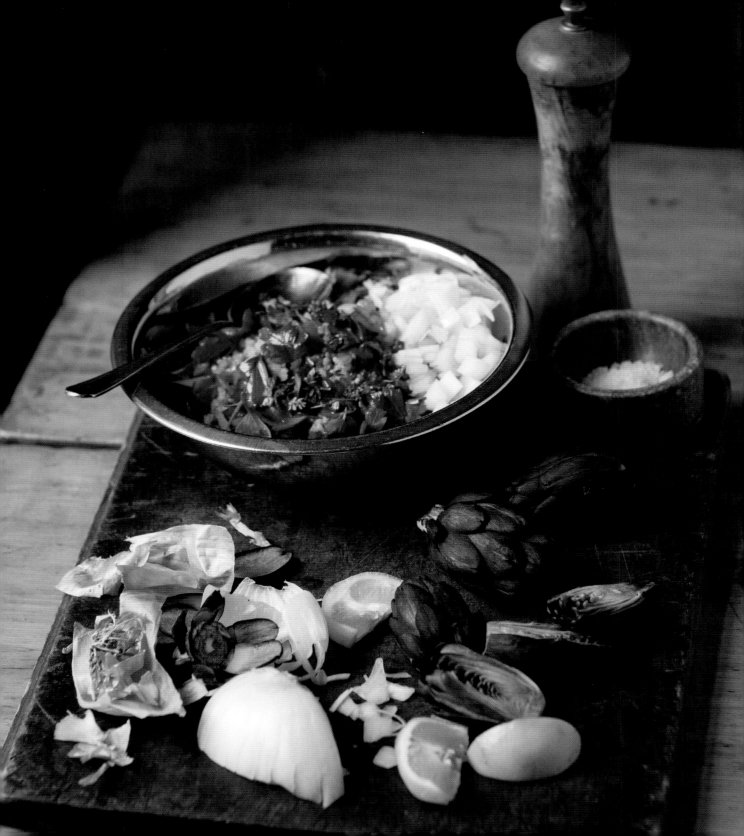

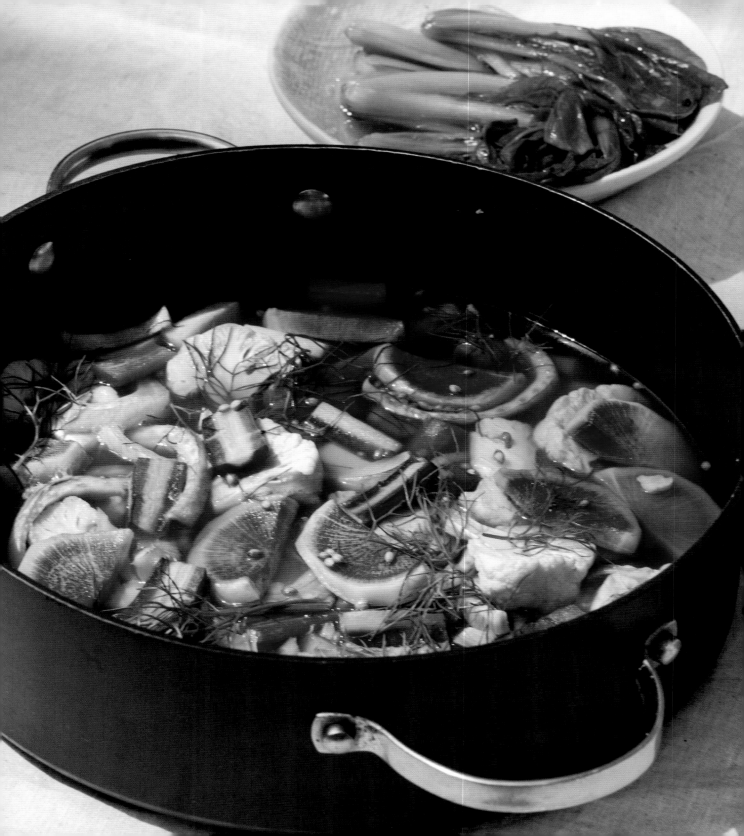

Bone Broth–Braised Winter Vegetables with Miso, Tahini, and Coconut

THIS VEGETABLE BRAISE IS ANOTHER RELIABLE OPTION IN A PINCH FOR THOSE NIGHTS WHEN there is little time to get dinner ready. Having bone broth at hand in the fridge can sometimes be a lifesaver! More than a recipe, this one is a tip—an idea for how to use bone broth to quickly cook flavorful vegetables and proteins, delivering a complete dinner on the table within minutes. Add any seasonings of your liking to the braising broth. If you would like to add protein, you could add whatever protein you have at hand, such as ground beef or lamb, pieces of roast chicken, cubed fish, sliced steak, cooked grains or beans, or even a couple of beaten eggs. Just remember to throw the densest vegetables in the pot first and allow them to soften a bit before adding more tender vegetables.

Yield: 4 servings

4 cups winter vegetables, such as sweet potatoes, potatoes, carrots, rutabaga, watermelon radish, and/or sunchokes, diced

1 quart beef, lamb, chicken, duck, or pork bone broth

1 heaping tablespoon cream of coconut

1 heaping tablespoon tahini (sesame paste)

1 heaping tablespoon good quality mild miso paste

1 tablespoon tamari sauce, nama shoyu sauce, or coconut amino acids

GARNISH

Chopped fresh herbs

1. Place the vegetables in a wide pot and pour the bone broth over to barely cover them (use less than 1 quart broth if necessary). Lower the heat and simmer until the vegetables soften. Check to make sure that the vegetables are always simmering in broth. If needed, add more broth or water to maintain the liquid level just barely covering the vegetables. Add the cream of coconut and mix well.

2. Once the coconut cream has dissolved and has been evenly incorporated into the braise, turn off the heat. Add the tahini and miso paste and stir well again.

3. Season to taste with tamari, shoyu, or aminos. A sprinkling of chopped fresh herbs would make a nice fresh final addition.

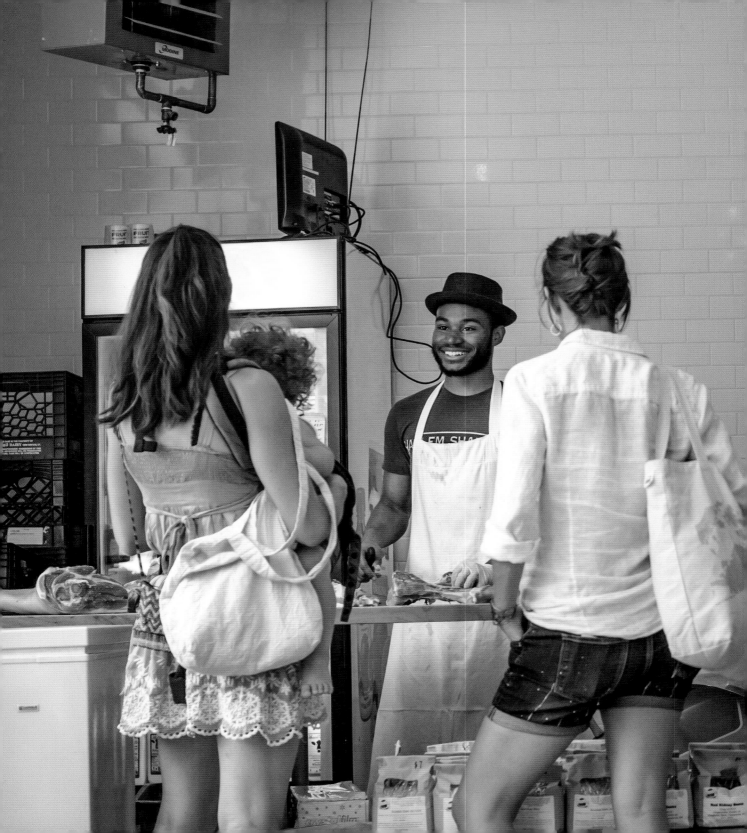

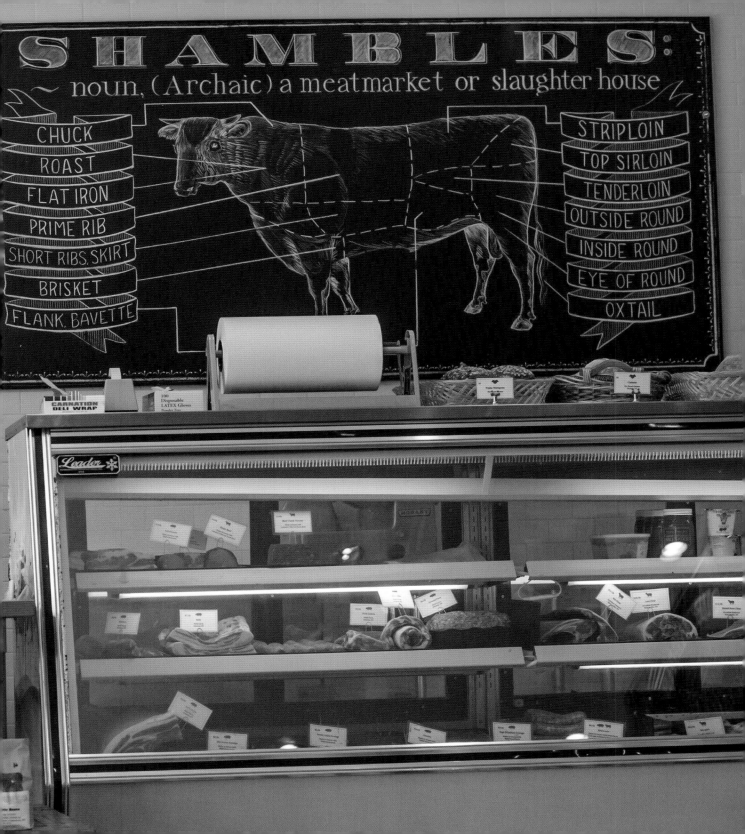

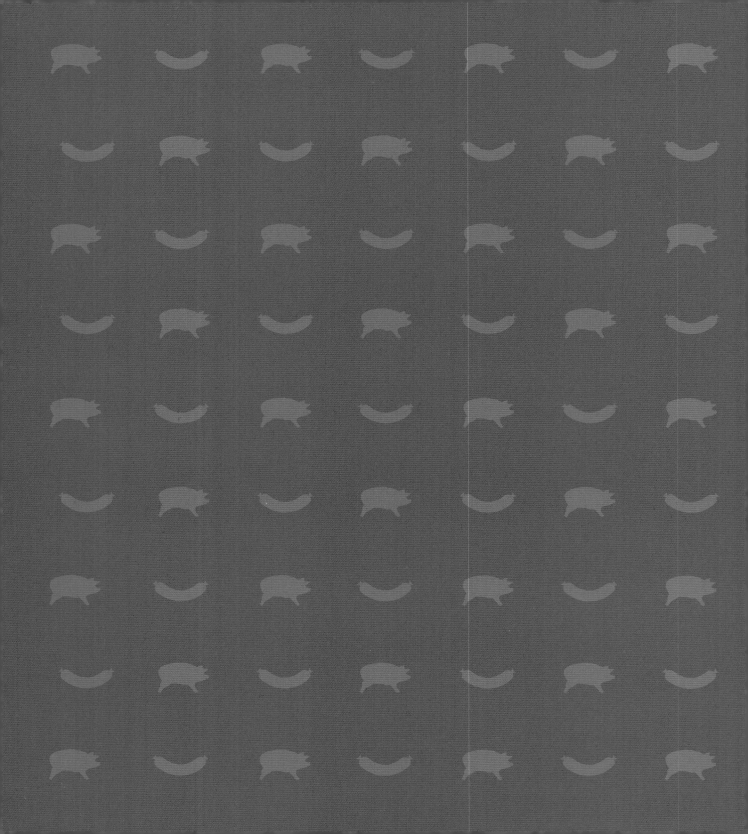

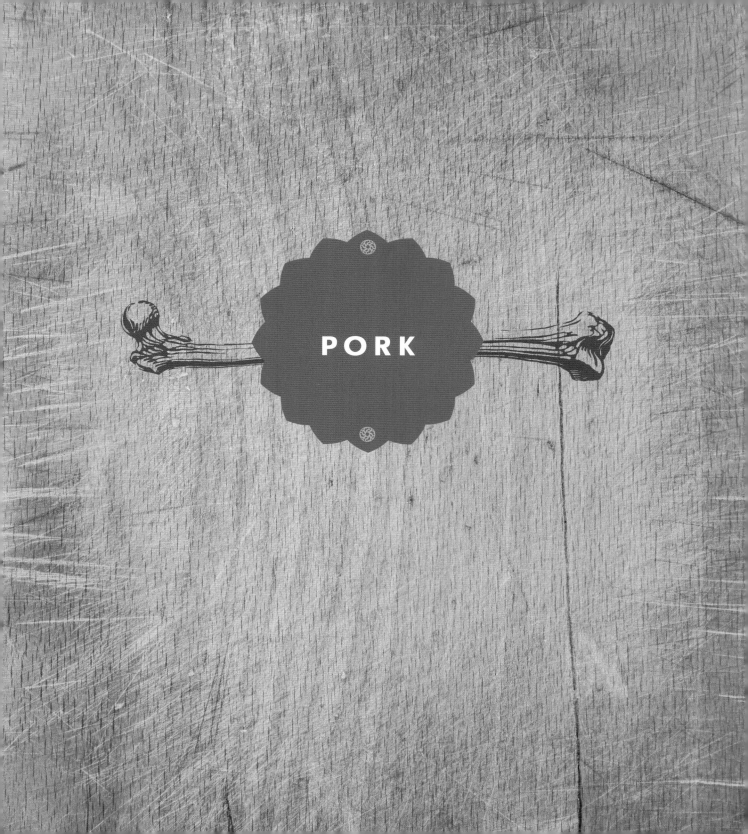

PORK

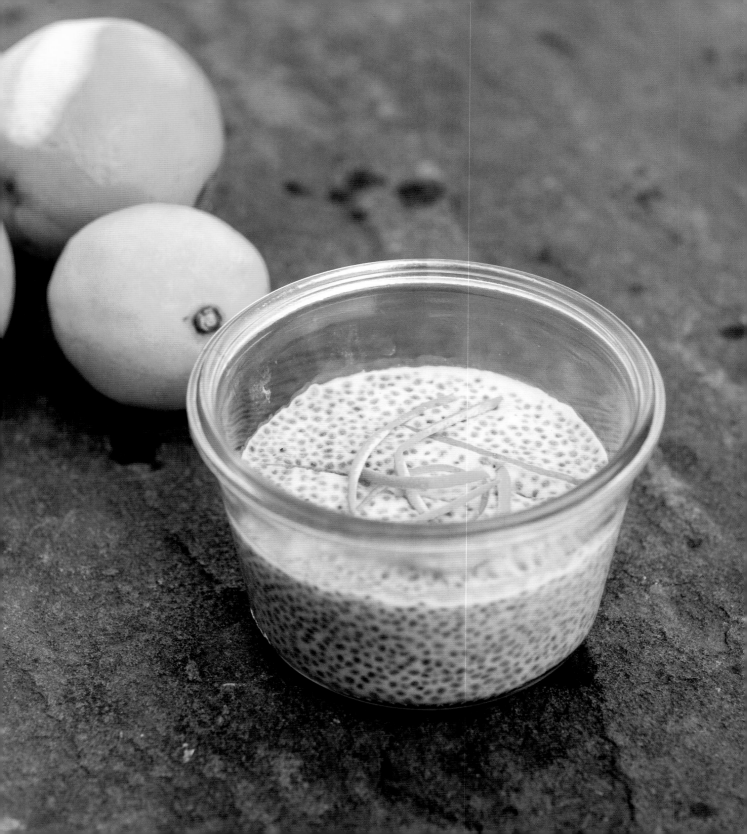

Bone Broth Chia Seed Pudding

AT BONE DEEP & HARMONY WE OCCASIONALLY RECEIVE REQUESTS FOR IDEAS
on how to incorporate bone broth into one's breakfast routine, without having to taste the broth. Oftentimes, this comes from longtime vegetarian or vegan customers who need more time adjusting to the broth flavor and idea of bone broth. By adding milk, honey, and citrus zest, the broth flavor becomes untraceable. This recipe may also be served as a healthful dessert.

Yield: 2 servings

1 cup beef or pork bone broth

¼ cup coconut or almond milk

Zest of 1 lemon or orange

1½ tablespoons honey or maple syrup

¼ cup chia seeds

1. Blend the bone broth, coconut or almond milk, citrus zest, and honey or maple syrup at high speed in a blender for about 1 minute. Turn the speed to the lowest level and gradually incorporate the chia seeds. You could also do all of this in a large bowl using a whisk, but it takes a little longer to achieve the desired smoothness.

2. Refrigerate for a few hours or overnight and serve.

Poached Eggs
in Tomato and Bone Broth Sauce

THIS RECIPE IS SIMPLE AND QUICK TO PREPARE. IT CAN BE THE FOUNDATION
for a richer and more complex dish if you add other vegetables, cheese, sausage,
or bacon to the eggs. We often make this for dinner when we get home late,
or when we don't have many ingredients in the fridge. It never disappoints!

Yield: 2 servings

3 tomatoes

Salt

½ tablespoon olive oil

1 cup beef or pork bone broth

1 clove garlic, minced

A few sprigs thyme (no stems) or
a pinch of oregano

Freshly ground black pepper

4 eggs

GARNISH

Fresh herbs, such as chives, parsley, mint, basil, or dill, chopped

1. Bring a small pot of water to a boil and add the tomatoes. When the skin of the tomatoes begins to break, remove them from the pot and place them in a colander. Run cold water over them or transfer to a bowl of ice water. You will be able to easily peel the skins off. Remove the cores, transfer two tomatoes to a blender, and blend with a pinch of salt. Chop the remaining tomato and set aside.

2. Warm the oil, preferably in a cast-iron pan. Add the blended tomatoes, chopped tomato, broth, garlic, and thyme or oregano. Bring to a boil, reduce the heat, and simmer for about 10 minutes. Season to taste with salt and pepper.

3. Crack the eggs into small separate bowls. Carefully transfer the eggs to the simmering sauce, one at a time. Continue to simmer just until the whites are cooked, about 3 minutes. Turn off the heat, and served topped with your choice of fresh chopped herbs.

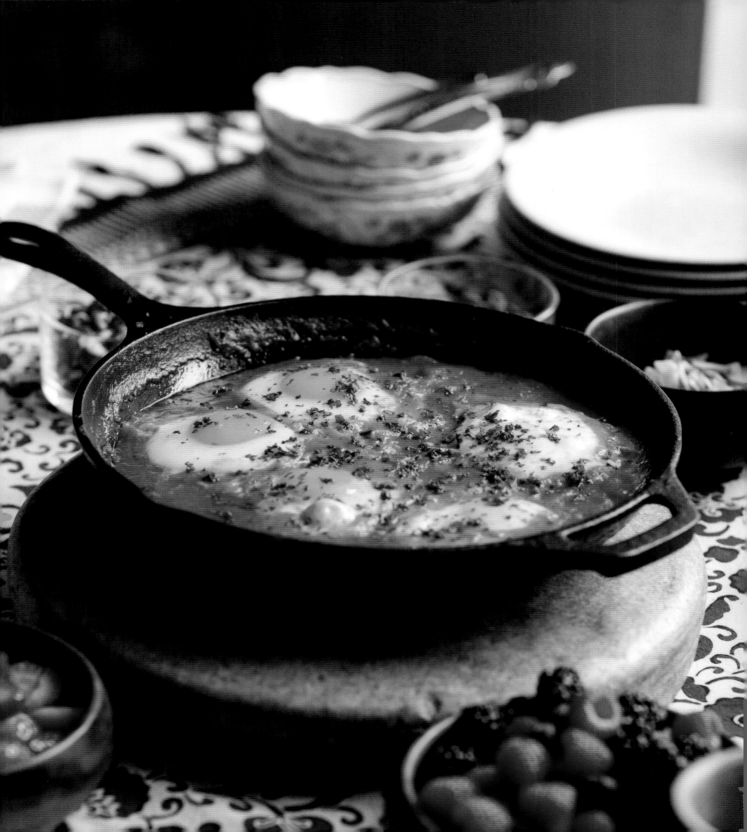

Pozole with Garbanzo Beans in Tomatillo and Pumpkin Seed Broth

POZOLE IS A TRADITIONAL MEXICAN SOUP OF HOMINY (CORN KERNELS THAT HAVE BEEN TREATED with an alkali solution) in a rich pork broth. Pozole is served with various garnishes including radishes, oregano, chili powder, avocado, lime, and small crispy tacos or tostadas (fried tortillas). There are various types of pozole: white, red, yellow, and green, determined by the color of the broth, which varies depending on the region in Mexico. Green pozole comes from the southern state of Guerrero, where Lya's grandfather was born. The green color of this broth comes from blended tomatillos and pumpkin seeds.

**If you cannot find tomatillos, substitute with tomatoes. We also use lard here, rendered from making pork broth. You can also substitute hominy with garbanzo beans, like we did in this recipe, for a corn-free dish.

Yield: 6–8 servings

1 cup pumpkin seeds (ideally pre-soaked, strained, dried, and lightly toasted) or store-bought sprouted pumpkin seeds

2 quarts pork bone broth, divided use

1 pound tomatillos, roughly chopped

3 serrano chiles or jalapeños, seeded and chopped

½ tablespoon lard

1 cup garbanzo beans (chickpeas), soaked for 24 hours, drained, rinsed, and cooked

GARNISHES
Shredded lettuce
Finely chopped onions
Crème fraîche
Crumbly fresh salty cheese, such as feta, cotija, or ricotta salata

1. In a food processor or blender, grind the pumpkin seeds. Mix the ground seeds with a little warmed pork broth and set aside.

2. Blend the tomatillos, chiles, and pumpkin seeds. Add a little more pork broth, if necessary, to form a smooth paste. Warm up the lard in a pot and fry the tomatillo sauce for 3 minutes. Add the rest of the pork broth and stir well. Bring to a boil, reduce the heat, add the cooked garbanzos, and simmer for 15 minutes.

3. Serve with your choice of garnishes.

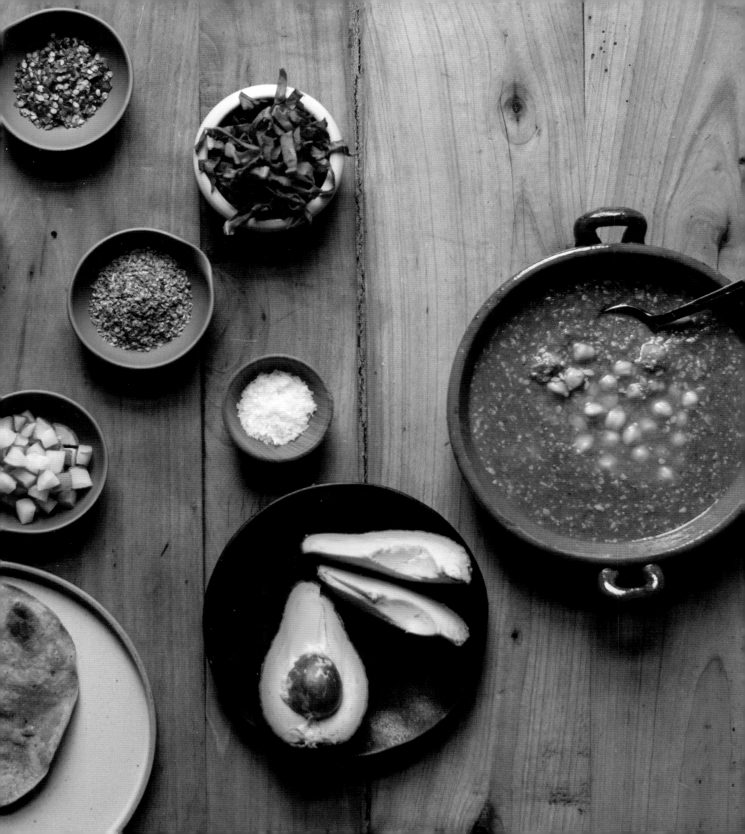

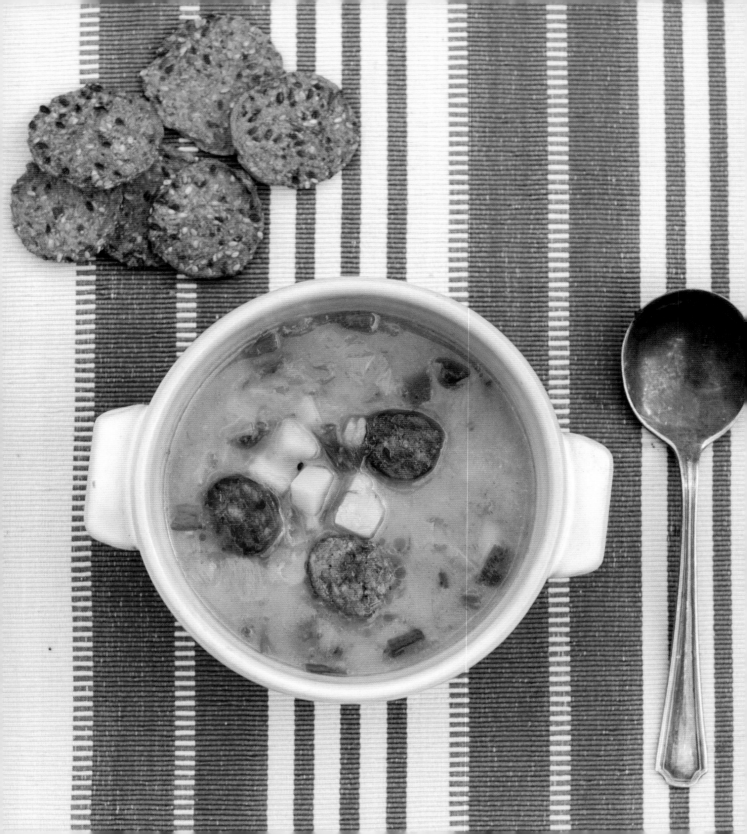

Caraway-Scented Potato, Leek, and Celery Soup with Chorizo

THIS IS A VERSION OF A CLASSIC COMFORT SOUP, WITH ENOUGH SUBSTANCE TO BE SERVED AS A main weekday meal. We like to top this soup with a few slices of chorizo for spice, texture, and added protein. In this recipe, caraway seed imparts a unique scent and flavor different from the classic soup. Caraway is similar in flavor to anise seed, which may be used as a substitute here.

Yield: 6 servings

¼ cup olive oil

2 large leeks, sliced

2 pounds potatoes, diced

2 celery stalks, sliced

6 cups pork bone broth

1 teaspoon caraway seeds

1 bay leaf

Salt and pepper to taste

1 handful cilantro or parsley

1 cup chorizo, sliced

1. Warm the olive oil over medium heat in a heavy-bottomed pot. Add the leeks and half-cover the pot to make the leeks sweat. When the leeks have reduced by half, add the potatoes and celery. Cook for 10 minutes.

2. Add the broth, caraway seeds, and bay leaf. Bring to a boil, reduce the heat, and simmer for 30 minutes.

3. Turn off the heat and allow to cool. After the soup cools down enough to handle, transfer 4 cups of it to a blender and purée. Return the blended soup to the pot. Season with salt and pepper to taste and add the chopped herbs. Cover the pot while you sauté the chorizo.

4. Warm a medium pan and brown the slices of chorizo on both sides. Ladle the soup into bowls and top with a few slices of chorizo.

Braised Mustard Greens and Leeks

TRADITIONALLY, THESE HEARTY MUSTARD GREENS ARE PREPARED WITH
butter and ham hocks, and Taylor's grandmother would say there's just no substitution
for classic collards over a mess of black-eyed peas and rice, with a dash of vinegar and
homemade chowchow. We like this variation on a classic Southern recipe.
Mustard greens have an especially sassy spice; paired with sweet leeks and braised in pork broth,
you've got quite a classy downtown dish with a hint of Southern charm.

Yield: 4 servings

2–4 leeks, depending on size

2 tablespoons unsalted butter

2 cups washed, dried, and chopped mustard greens (1 large bunch)

½ cup pork bone broth (can easily substitute chicken or beef broth)

Salt and ground black pepper to taste

2 tablespoons grated Parmesan cheese

1. Trim the leeks so that about 1½ inches of green leaves remain, and slice the leeks in half lengthwise. Separate the leaves and pull the leeks apart to rinse away any dirt and sand in the layers, then chop them into 1½ inch pieces.

2. Melt the butter in a skillet over medium heat. Cook the leeks, stirring, until they begin to separate and soften, about 5 minutes.

3. Stir in the mustard greens and pour in enough broth to just cover the bottom of the pan and prevent the leeks from browning. Cook the leeks and mustard greens until the greens turn bright green and start to soften, another 2–3 minutes. Season to taste with salt and black pepper, and sprinkle with Parmesan cheese.

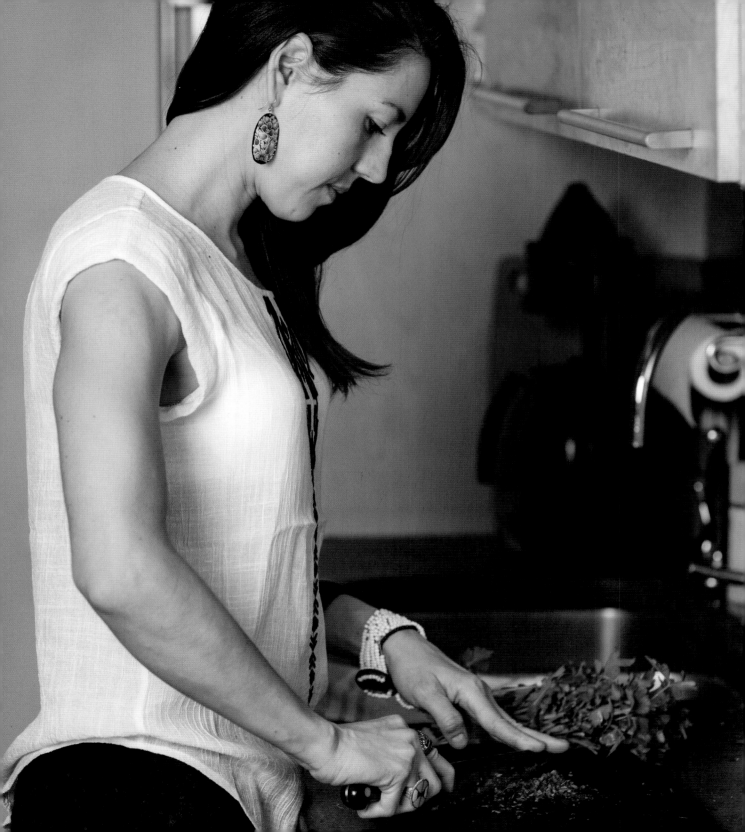

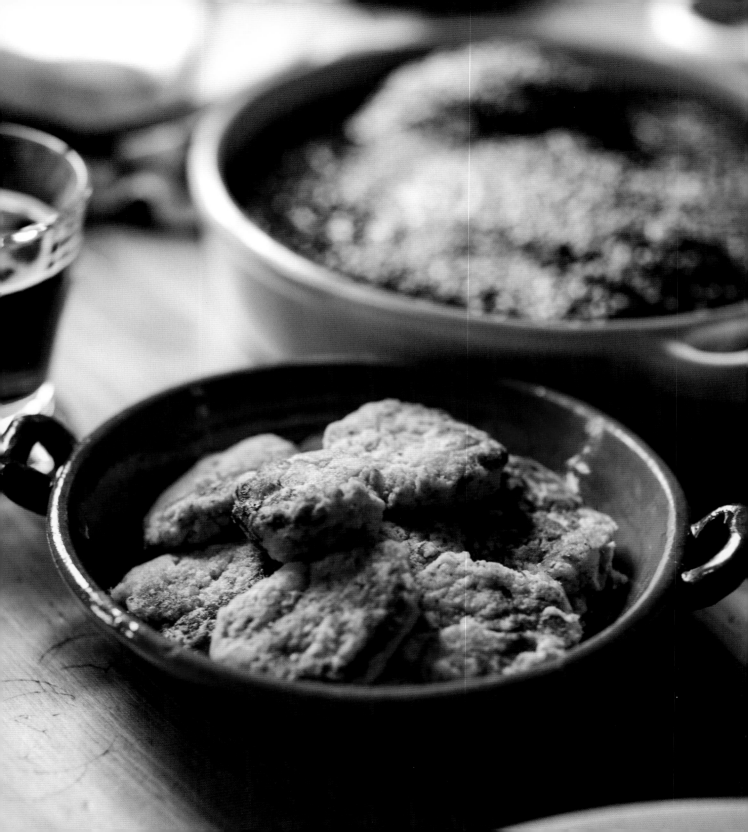

Tortitas:
Sweet Potato, Plantain, and Bone Broth Fritters

INSPIRED BY A CHILDHOOD FAVORITE OF LITTLE POTATO FRITTERS MADE WITH MILK AND butter, we created a revised version using Japanese sweet potato, plantain, and bone broth. The binding agents here are egg yolk and coconut flour. Japanese sweet potato is white on the inside, and is somewhat sweeter than regular sweet potatoes, but any sweet potato will do. This is a great recipe for those on dairy and grain-free diets, and a delicious starchy accompaniment to meals.

Yield: 10–12 tortitas

1 pound Japanese sweet potatoes (about 2 small)

1 tablespoon coconut oil or lard, plus more for frying the tortitas

1 green plantain sliced in ¾ inch pieces

¾ cup pork bone broth

2 tablespoons coconut flour

1 egg yolk

1 teaspoon salt

1 whole nutmeg

1. Using a fork or a paring knife, prick each potato a few times all around. Fill a medium pot with water and bring to a boil. Add the potatoes, lower the heat, and half-cover the pot. Cook the potatoes until soft.

2. In the meantime, warm 1 tablespoon coconut oil in a skillet and sauté the plantain slices until golden on both sides. Transfer to a plate lined with paper towels to remove excess oil. Mash the plantains with a fork.

3. In a separate small pot, bring the broth to a boil and turn off the heat.

4. While the bone broth cools a little, drain, peel, and mash the sweet potatoes with a fork. Add the mashed plantains and slightly cooled bone broth. Mix well. Incorporate the coconut flour, egg yolk, and salt. Using a fine grater, add 5 or 6 gratings of nutmeg. Combine everything well.

5. Using your hands, form golf ball–sized tortitas. Warm a little more coconut oil or lard in a skillet and fry the tortitas on each side until golden. Be cautious when transferring the uncooked tortitas to the skillet, as they are very soft. Fry them in small batches for easier handling.

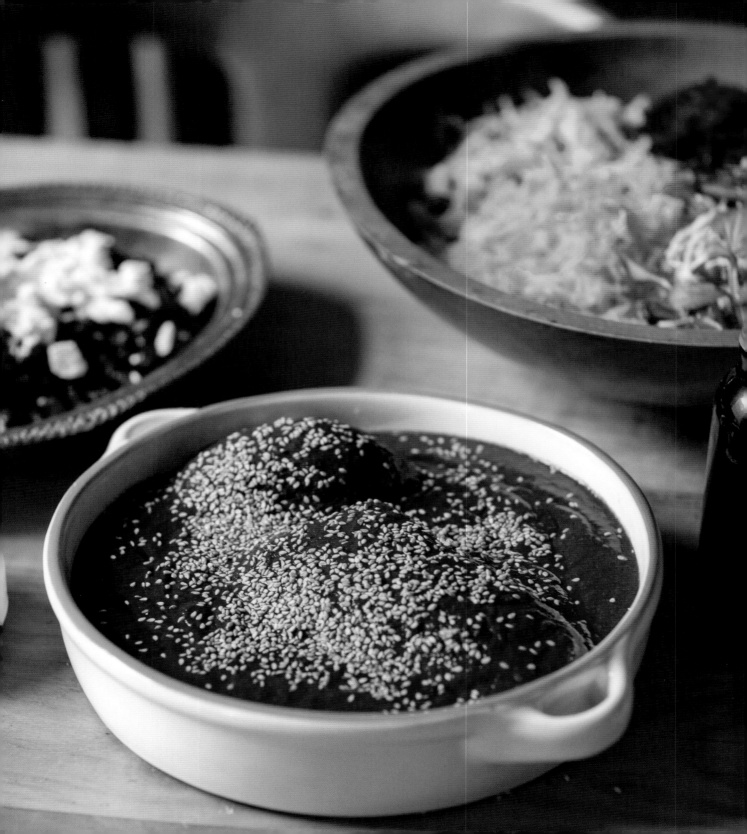

"One of the things that brought me into Chinese medicine was the desire to learn how to manage my own autoimmune disease. One of the pillars in the treatment of autoimmune disease is ensuring that the body's belly is fully functioning; when my belly is off, I'm off, more so than most people. When I'm able to regularly consume bone broth, my antibodies decrease, my gut permeability decreases, and I'm actually able to get nutrients out of my food. It's something I rely on to help manage my body's response system."

—*Heidi Lovie,*
LICENSED NEW YORK CITY ACUPUNCTURIST

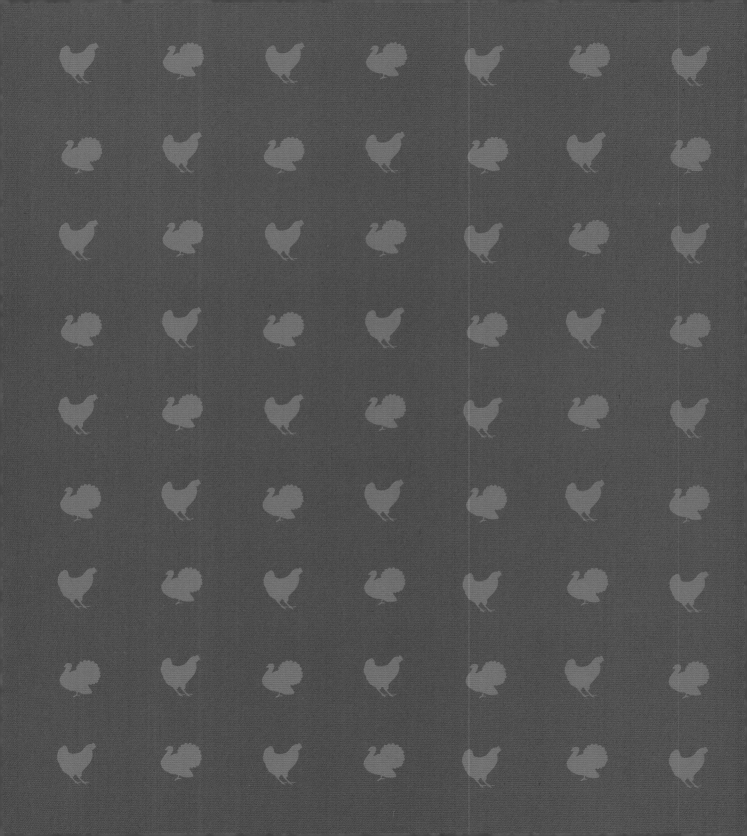

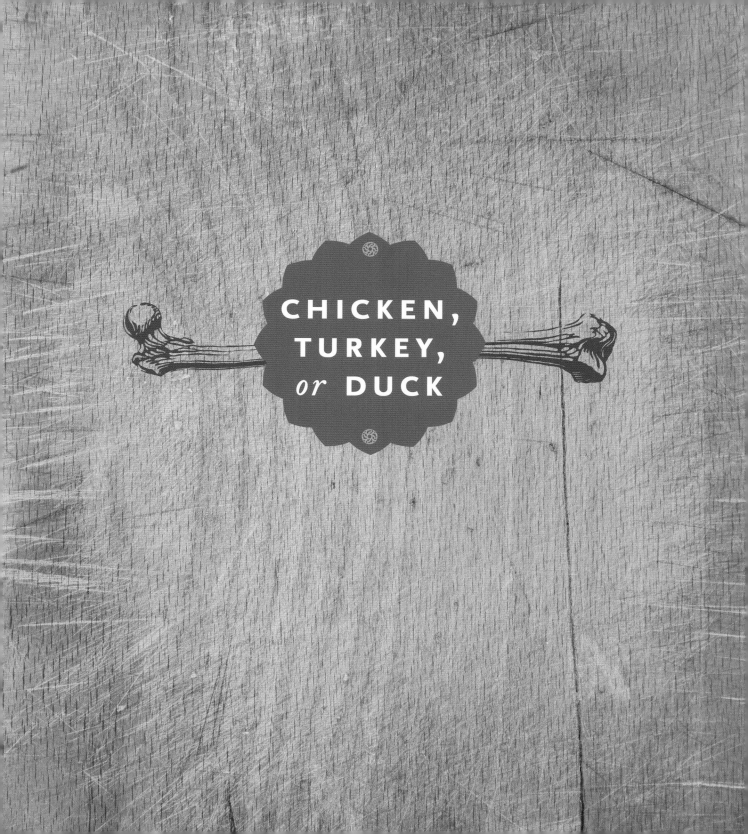

CHICKEN, TURKEY, *or* **DUCK**

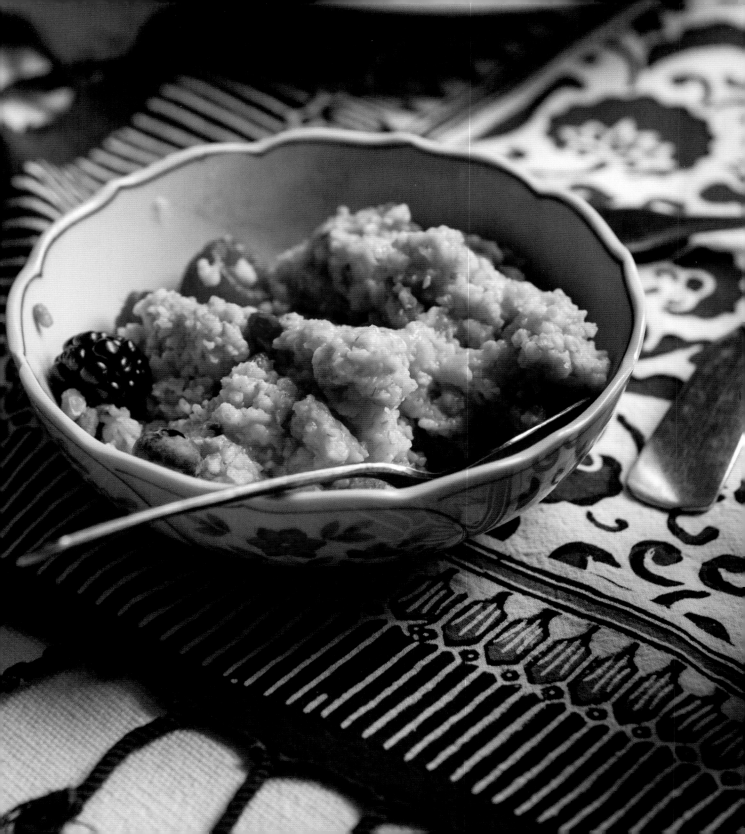

Breakfast Oatmeal Porridge

BROTH FINDS ITS WAY INTO UNUSUAL PLACES IN OUR HOMES. THIS OATMEAL IS one of them, and it's become one of our family's favorite breakfasts. Feel free to substitute with any available nuts, seeds, and dried or fresh fruits. Ideally, soak the oats, nuts, and seeds the night before, to optimize nutrient absorption. In this recipe, we use whole cloves and cardamom. These two spices are water-soluble, meaning that they release their flavor efficiently in a liquid base, which is ideal for this recipe. If you choose to use a ground version of these spices, we recommend that you grind the spices right before using.

Yield: 4 servings

1 cup steel cut oats

1½ cups water

1 tablespoon acidic liquid, such as yogurt, kefir, buttermilk, vinegar, or lemon juice

1 cup beef or chicken bone broth

1 pinch salt

1 teaspoon cinnamon

2 cloves

2 cardamom pods

¼ cup goji berries

2 tablespoons dried cherries

Butter (preferably cultured and from grass-fed cows)

Toasted pine nuts

Toasted coconut flakes, unsweetened

1. Soak the oatmeal overnight in the water and acidic liquid.

2. Strain and rinse the oatmeal from the overnight soak. Transfer to a pot with the broth, salt, cinnamon, cloves, and cardamom pods. Bring to a boil, reduce the heat, and add the goji berries and cherries. Cover and simmer gently until the broth is absorbed into the oats and the oats are cooked through. The overnight soaking of the oats shortens the cooking time to about 10 minutes. Remove the cloves and cardamom pods after cooking.

3. Serve with a pat of butter and top with toasted pine nuts and coconut flakes.

GRAINS AND PORRIDGES

Grains, legumes, nuts, and seeds contain phytic acid. When we consume foods that have phytic acid, the acid binds important minerals like calcium, magnesium, zinc, and iron in the intestines. When these minerals are bound, we are not able to assimilate them. Soaking, sprouting, and fermenting are ancient techniques that reduce the amount of phytic acid by releasing enzymes that help break down and neutralize it. In these recipes, the added nutritional benefit of cooking grains in bone broth is that the gelatin in the broth further facilitates digestion, as well as providing more of the important minerals that may be lost to phytates in the grains.

Egg Drop Soup with Spinach Ribbons

MANY A MORNING IN OUR HOMES BEGINS WITH AN EGG CRACKED INTO A BOWL OF piping hot broth, often with spicy kimchi and a dash of sesame oil. Hello happy gut, clear sinuses, and smooth energy! What we love most is the simplicity of these soups and the endless possibility for variation. This classic Italian recipe, usually called *stracciatella,* always strikes us like our favorite style icons: elegant, put together, and fuss-free, with just a hint of mystique.

Yield: 4 servings

5 cups chicken bone broth

Salt

4 large eggs

½ teaspoon nutmeg

Zest of 1 lemon, grated

Freshly ground black pepper

¼ cup Parmesan cheese, grated, divided use

1 cup shredded spinach

2–3 tablespoons chopped Italian parsley

1. In a soup pot over high heat, bring the broth to a boil. Season to taste with salt and reduce the heat to a simmer.

2. Crack the eggs into a medium bowl and beat lightly with a wire whisk. Whisk in the nutmeg, the lemon zest, a large pinch of salt, several twists of the pepper mill, and 2 tablespoons Parmesan. Add the shredded spinach to the broth, then pour in the egg mixture and whisk gently until the egg mixture forms *stracciatella* ("little rags"). Simmer 1 additional minute.

3. Ladle the soup into individual bowls and garnish with parsley, fresh pepper, and the remaining Parmesan.

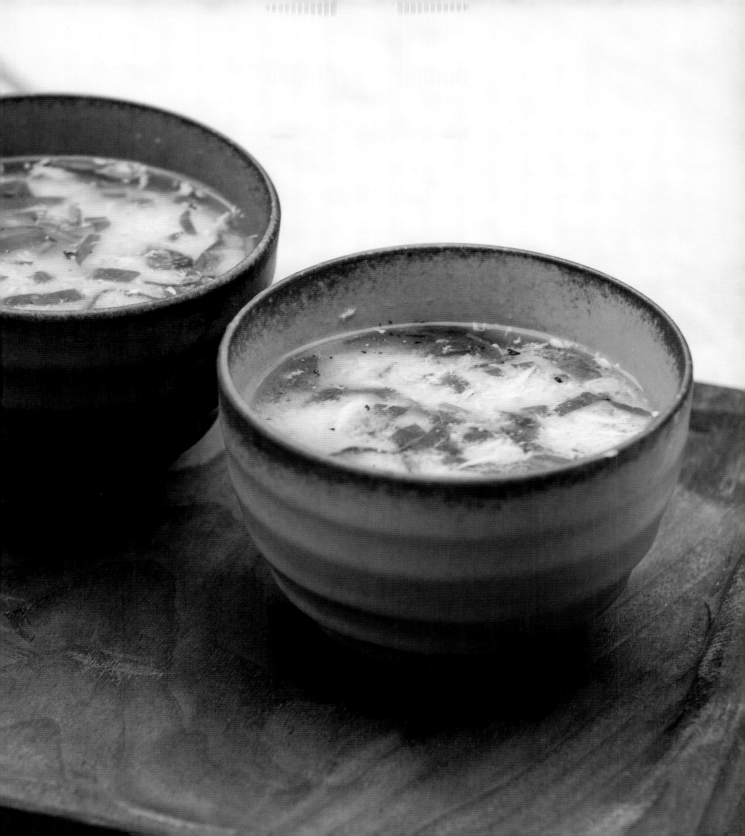

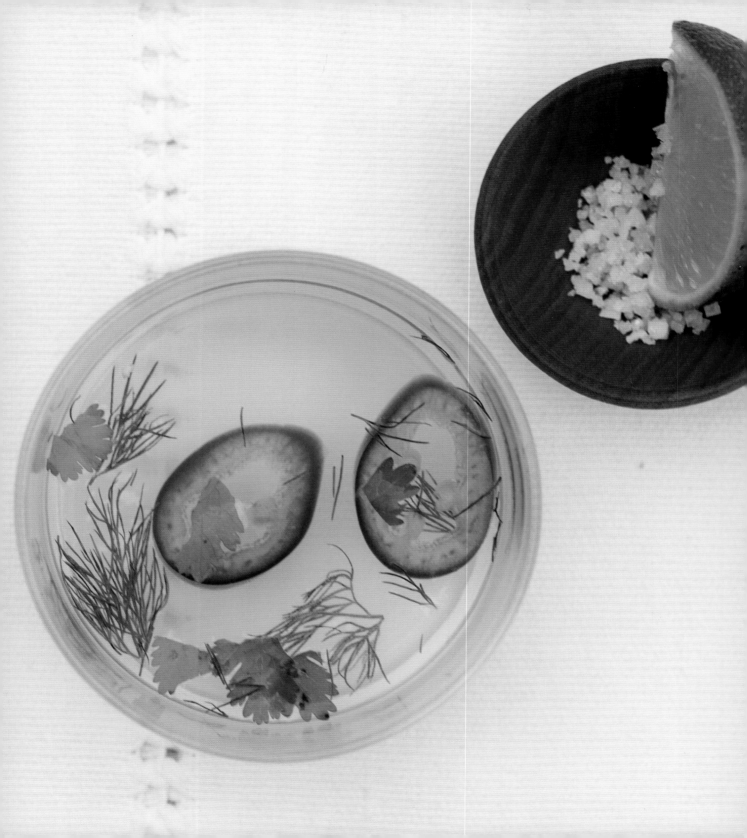

Tequila Consommé

CONSOMMÉ IS TRADITIONALLY SERVED AT THE BEGINNING OF MEALS IN DIFFERENT CULTURES around the world, including the Spanish, French, and some Latin American cultures. It opens up the palate for the meal to come, and prepares the digestive system to receive food. Consommé is delicate and light as a result of clarification. The process of clarification removes any solids left in the broth after it has been strained from the bones and aromatics for a cleaner mouthfeel. The clarifying agents used here are egg whites with a little acid from the tomatoes.

Yield: 8 servings

2 quarts chicken or duck bone broth

4 egg whites, lightly beaten

1 leek, chopped

2 tomatoes, peeled and chopped

½ cup tequila

Julienned vegetables (your choice)

Fresh chopped herbs (your choice)

1. Bring the broth to a quick boil. Add the egg whites, leek, and tomatoes, stirring constantly. Reduce the heat to a simmer, and simmer for 30 minutes, stirring occasionally.

2. Remove from the heat and strain through a fine-mesh colander lined with a couple of layers of cheesecloth.

3. Return the clarified broth to the pot, and bring to a quick boil again. Reduce the heat and add the tequila. Simmer gently for 5 minutes. Add the julienned vegetables and simmer for 3–5 minutes more. Serve immediately, adding fresh chopped herbs of your choice.

Chicken Congee
with Sweet Potato, Shiitake, and Ginger

"CONGEE," OR "JOOK" IS SIMPLY A TRADITIONAL RICE PORRIDGE COMMONLY EATEN FOR breakfast or any meal. There are many varieties ranging from sweet or savory, to herbal and medicinal. To make the porridge as gentle on the system as possible, the rice is usually blended, yielding a soupy consistency when cooked. If using this recipe for entertaining, we think the dish looks prettier with the full grain rice and slightly less broth. Just disregard the first step! You can also eliminate the chicken for a nourishing "meatless" meal.

Yield: 4 servings

1 cup short-grain brown rice or sweet sticky rice, soaked overnight, rinsed, and drained

1 cup water

1 tablespoon unrefined organic coconut oil

2 garlic cloves, thinly sliced

1 thumb-sized piece ginger root, minced (we often double this for a good zing)

1 cup sliced fresh or dried shiitake mushrooms (if using dried, presoak in hot water for 20 minutes)

2 chicken thighs

2 chicken drumsticks

1 cup diced sweet potato

3 cups chicken bone broth

Salt or soy sauce

White or black pepper

1. Combine the presoaked rice with the water in the blender and blend on the low setting for 10 seconds.

2. Heat the oil in a large, heavy pot over medium heat. Sauté the garlic, ginger, and mushrooms until the mushrooms are softened.

3. Add the chicken, rice, sweet potato, and broth and bring to a boil. Reduce to a simmer and cook, stirring occasionally to prevent the rice from sticking to the bottom. Simmer covered for 1 hour or until the rice has absorbed most of the liquid and the chicken is well cooked.

4. Remove chicken thighs from the pot and allow to cool. When cool enough to handle, shred the chicken meat and skin and discard the bones.

5. Add the shredded meat back into the congee.

6. Continue simmering for another 30 minutes or so until it reaches the consistency of porridge. Cook to your own preference; some people prefer it more soupy, others thicker. Season to taste with salt or soy sauce and pepper. Serve hot with the garnishes and condiments of your choice.

**GARNISHES AND CONDIMENTS
(YOUR CHOICE)**

Soft-boiled egg

Thinly sliced scallions

Chopped fresh cilantro

Chopped roasted almonds

Toasted quinoa

Sesame seeds

Soy sauce

Sesame oil

Fish sauce

Chili paste

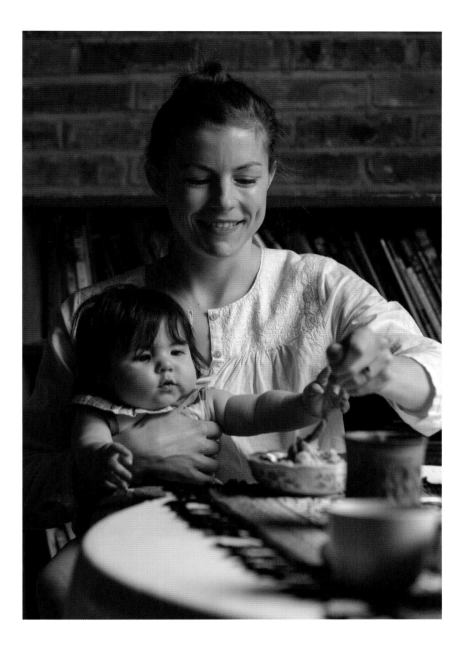

7. Congee may be refrigerated for a few days, but the consistency will become thicker. Add more water or stock when reheating.

Late Summer Corn Soup
with Roasted Peppers

IN AUGUST, WE END UP WITH AN ABUNDANCE OF EARS OF SWEET CORN
from our CSA share (Community Supported Agriculture). With poblano peppers
also making an appearance at farmers markets around this time, it's a match made in heaven.
This soup is one of our favorite (and easiest) ways to use some of the late summer bounty.

Yield: 6 servings

2 poblano peppers (substitute bell peppers if you prefer a non-spicy soup)

1 tablespoon coconut or olive oil

1 onion, chopped

1 teaspoon fresh oregano

1 teaspoon fresh thyme

4 ears corn, kernels removed from the cobs, cobs broken in half and reserved

6 cups chicken or pork bone broth

1 small handful cilantro, chopped

Salt and pepper to taste

1. Over an open flame on your stove or under the broiler, roast the peppers, turning constantly with tongs, until they turn black all around. Place them in a bowl, cover them, and set them aside.

2. In a large, heavy-bottomed pot, heat the oil. Sauté the onions with the oregano and thyme. When the onions are very soft, after about 10 minutes, add the corn kernels and sauté for another 5–10 minutes. Add the broth and the reserved cobs. Bring to a boil, reduce heat, and simmer for 20–30 minutes to blend the flavors.

3. In the meantime, rub off the burned skin of the peppers (it's easy if you use a paper towel). Discard the seeds and the cores of the peppers and chop the flesh. Remove the soup from the heat, discard the cobs, and allow the soup to cool a little.

4. Using a slotted spoon, skim out about half of the corn kernels; set aside. Blend the soup until creamy. Return the reserved kernels to the soup along with the roasted peppers and cilantro. Season with salt and pepper to taste.

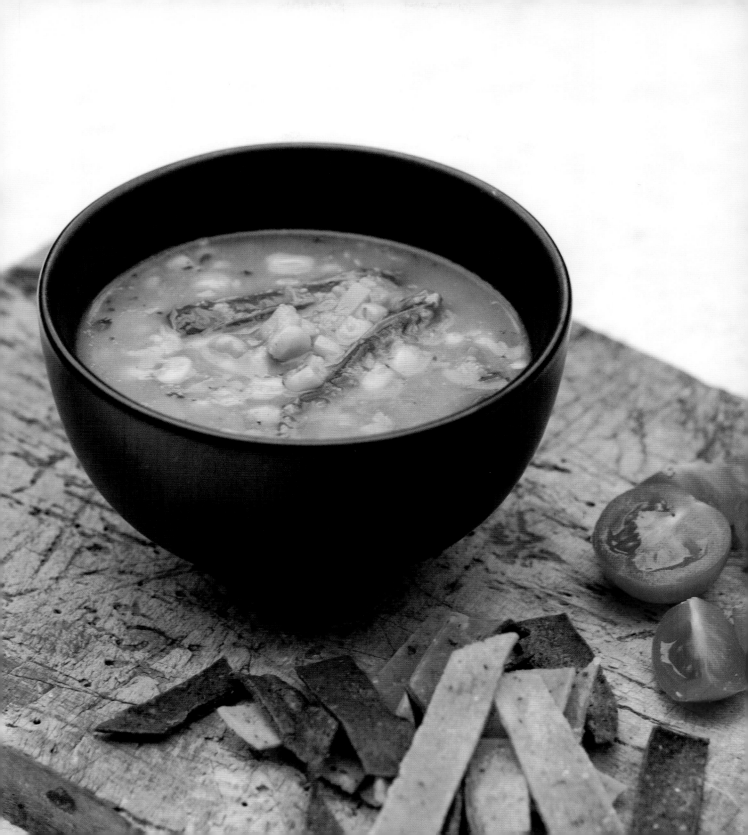

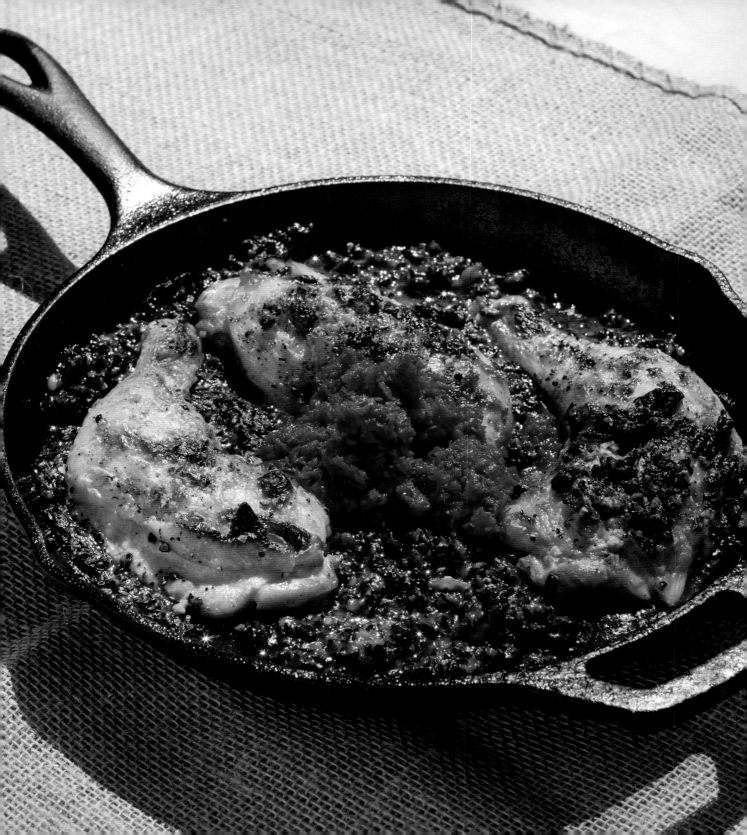

Arroz Negro con Pollo

THIS IS OUR DOLLED-UP VERSION OF A BASIC ARROZ CON POLLO, A FAVORITE GO-TO FOR A summer supper or family-style meal. Substituting black rice for white adds not only nutritional value, but dramatic effect, especially when topped with bright pink beet horseradish and fresh cilantro. Pair with a bright and crunchy salad and crisp cold beers or fresh margaritas, and enjoy!

**There is always ample leftover rice when making this dish.
Re-purpose it by adding any mix of additional vegetables, diced avocado, scallion, and/or a poached egg for the next day's breakfast or lunch.

**Curtido is a traditional Latin American fermented salad similar to kimchi or sauerkraut. It can be found at most Latin supermarkets.

Yield: 2 servings

¾ cup pickled peppers or curtido

2 tablespoons coconut oil

2 chicken thighs

2 chicken drumsticks

Flaked salt, such as Maldon

Fresh ground black pepper

½ tablespoon cumin

1½ cups presoaked black rice

4 cups chicken bone broth

3 tablespoons beet horseradish (recipe p. 118)

Fresh cilantro leaves

1. In a small blender, blend the pickled peppers until coarsely chopped. If using curtido, there is no need to blend.

2. Heat the oil over medium-high heat in cast-iron pot. Coat the chicken generously with flaked salt, pepper, and cumin. Add the chicken to the pot and sear to crisp skin, about 2 minutes each side.

3. Remove the chicken and add the pickled peppers to the pot. Cook over medium heat until they gently caramelize.

4. Add the rice and broth to the pot, bring to a boil, and then reduce heat to simmer. Add the chicken on top. Cover and cook over medium heat until the rice and chicken are fully cooked, about 45 minutes.

5. Plate and serve with a dollop of beet horseradish and fresh cilantro.

(Continued)

2 medium beets

4 ounces fresh horseradish, peeled

¼ cup cider vinegar

2 teaspoons salt

1 teaspoon sugar

BEET HORSERADISH

Yield: roughly 1 cup

1. Scrub the beets; cut off the greens and reserve for sautéing as a side or using in a salad. Place the beets in a medium saucepan; add water to cover by 1 inch. Bring to a boil over high heat.

2. Reduce the heat to medium-high; cook at a gentle boil until the beets are tender when pierced with a small, sharp knife, 30–40 minutes.

3. Remove from the heat, drain, and set aside until the beets are cool enough to handle.

4. Meanwhile, grate the horseradish on the small holes of a box grater. Place in a small bowl and stir in the vinegar, salt, and sugar.

5. Peel the beets and grate on the small holes of box grater. Add to the horse-radish mixture and stir well to combine. Jar and refrigerate until needed.

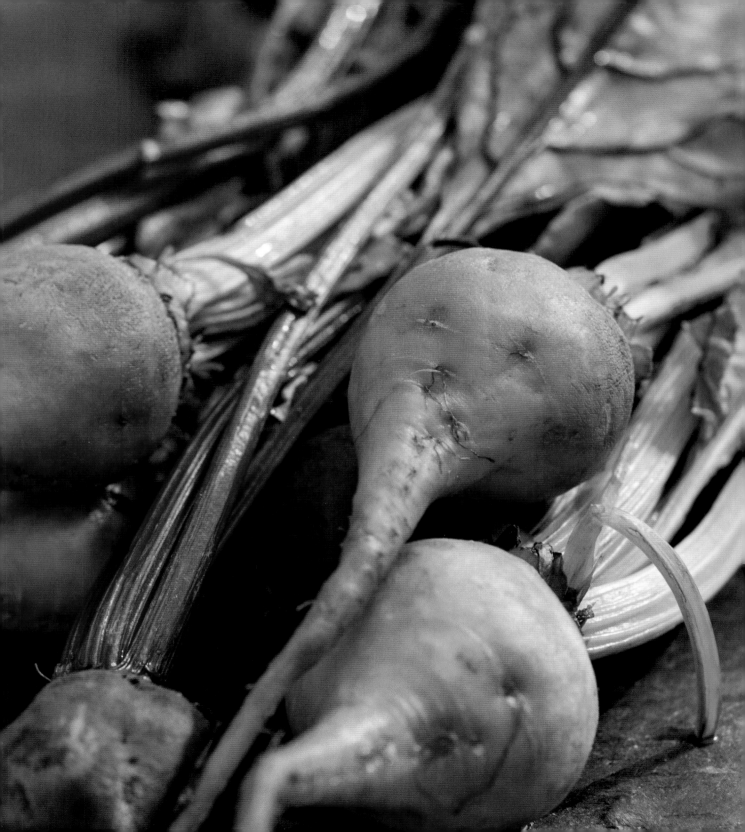

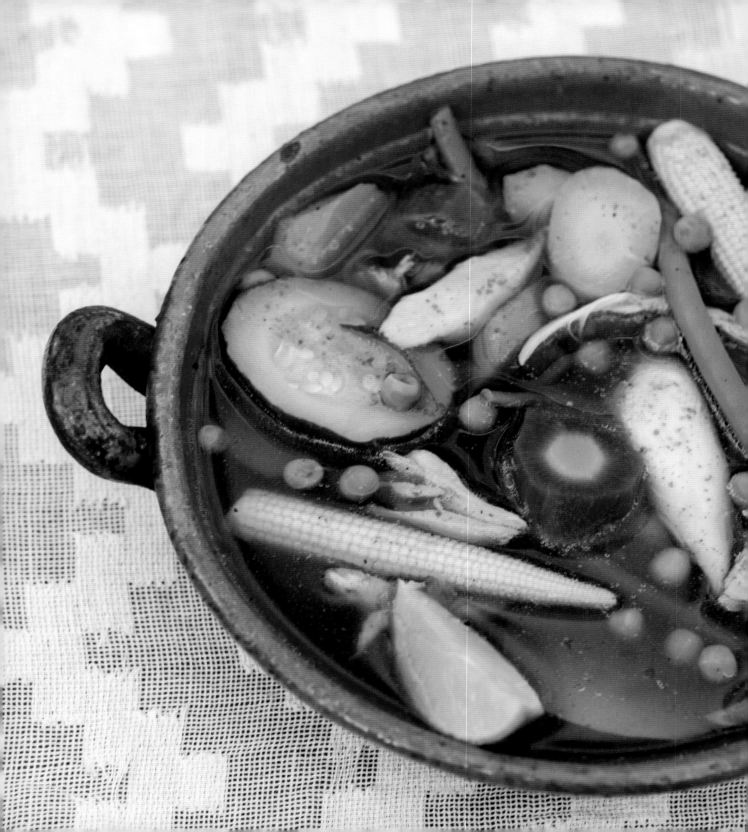

Gloria's Mole de Olla

MOLE DE OLLA IS AN UNPRETENTIOUS EVERYDAY MEXICAN SOUP: BONE BROTH BLENDED with roasted pasilla and ancho chiles, tomatoes, and cumin. This soup is commonly served with big chunks of vegetables and pieces of chicken or beef. Gloria, Lya's family cook in Mexico, prepared this soup once a week for lunch. We accompanied it with steaming hot tortillas and a wedge of lime. Sometimes, we added spoonfuls of rice and pinto beans.

Yield: 4 servings

2 dried ancho chiles

2 dried pasilla chiles (also called chile negro)

3 tomatoes, peeled and quartered

1 pinch cumin seeds

2 tablespoons lard, tallow, or olive oil

Bite-size pieces of poached or roasted chicken, or slices of steak

6 cups chicken bone broth

Seasonal vegetables: 2 cups, cubed (in Mexico the soup is most often made with green beans, zucchini, chayote squash, slices of corn on the cob, and potato)

1. Dry-roast the ancho and pasilla chiles until fragrant. Remove the seeds and stems and blend in a blender with the tomatoes and cumin seeds.

2. In a heavy-bottomed deep pot, fry the chile paste in lard, tallow, or olive oil. After 3–5 minutes, add the chicken or steak and mix thoroughly. Add the broth and bring to a quick boil. Reduce the heat, add the vegetables, and simmer until the vegetables are cooked but not too soft.

Chipotle- and Cumin-Scented Farro and Vegetable Soup

ON WEEKNIGHTS, WE FAVOR SIMPLE MEALS LIKE THIS SOUP.
The trick is that we prepare a huge batch of bone broth once a month,
so that we can pull it out of our refrigerators or freezers on any given night.
If you prefer, substitute the farro or spelt berries with quinoa for a gluten-free meal.

Yield: 4–6 servings

½ tablespoon coconut oil

1 onion, chopped

1 whole dried chipotle chile

1 teaspoon cumin seeds

2 celery stalks, chopped

2 carrots, sweet potatoes, or any winter squash, diced

1 cup red or green cabbage, chopped

¾ cup farro or spelt berries, soaked for at least 12 hours, strained, and rinsed

2 quarts chicken bone broth

Salt and pepper to taste

Sauerkraut or any pickled vegetable

Parsley or cilantro, chopped

1. In a heavy-bottomed pot, heat the oil and sauté the onion with the chipotle and cumin seeds until the onions begin to soften. Add the celery and carrots (or sweet potatoes or winter squash), and stir to mix all the ingredients thoroughly. When the carrots soften a little, 3–5 minutes, add the cabbage and farro or spelt, and mix well one more time. Remove the chipotle chile at this point for a less spicy soup, otherwise keep it. Add the bone broth and bring to a boil. Reduce the heat, half-cover the pot, and simmer for 45–60 minutes, or until the farro is fully cooked. If you didn't do so before, remove the chipotle chile now. Add more bone broth or water along the way if necessary.

2. Season to taste. Garnish with sauerkraut and chopped parsley or cilantro.

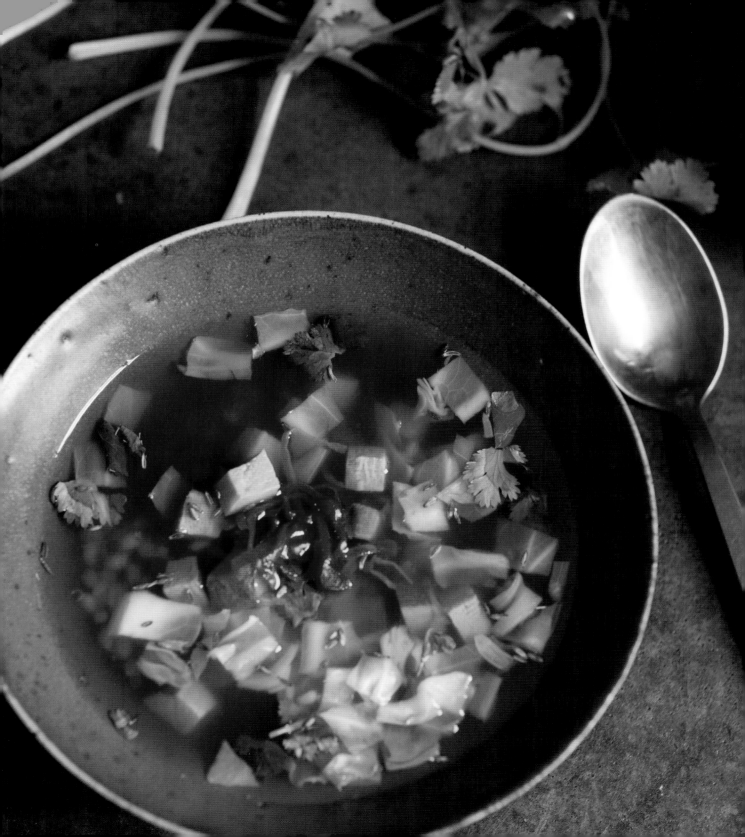

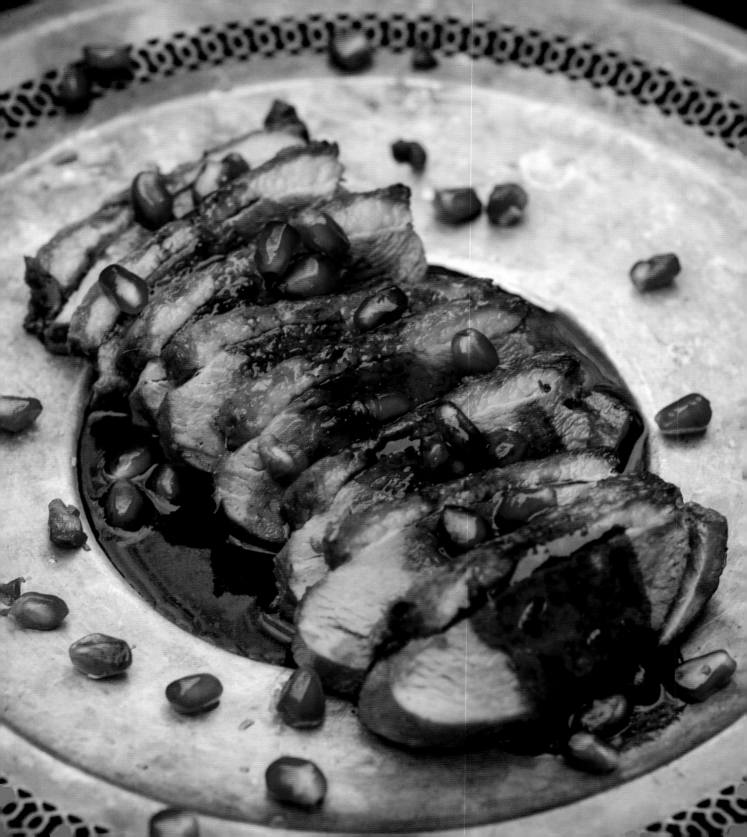

Roasted Duck
with Pomegranate, Balsamic,
and Bone Broth Sauce

THE RICHNESS OF THE DUCK MEAT IS BRIGHTENED BY THE TANGINESS OF THE BALSAMIC and pomegranate in this dish. This is a very easy recipe to make, but it sounds and looks fancy. It would make a nice dinner party main dish. If you are able to find fresh pomegranates, reserve some of the seeds for garnish. The stunning contrast between the black colored sauce and the bright red seeds will wow your guests!

Yield: 4 servings

2 duck breasts

Salt and pepper

½ cup balsamic vinegar

Juice of 2 pomegranates or 1 cup store-bought pomegranate juice

⅔ cup chicken or duck bone broth

1 tablespoon butter

Fresh pomegranate seeds

1. Score the skin side of the duck breasts, making diagonal cuts in opposite directions to form diamond shapes. Rub them all over with salt and pepper.

2. In an oven-proof medium pan (preferably cast iron), sear the duck skin side down until golden, about 3–5 minutes. Flip the duck and sear for 5 minutes more for medium-rare or 8 minutes for medium. Transfer the duck to a cutting board. Let it rest for a few minutes while you prepare the sauce.

3. Discard the excess fat from the pan. Over medium-high heat, deglaze the pan with the balsamic vinegar. Reduce by half. Add the pomegranate juice and reduce by half again. Add the bone broth, bring to a boil, turn the heat down, and reduce by half one more time. Season to taste with salt and pepper. Swirl the butter in, and remove from the heat immediately. Leave the sauce undisturbed for a few minutes. It will thicken and acquire a syruplike consistency.

4. Slice the duck and serve drizzled with the sauce and sprinkled with fresh pomegranate seeds.

Mole

MOLE IS AN ANCIENT MEXICAN SAUCE OF SOPHISTICATED COMPLEXITY. IT COMBINES A VARIETY of flavors from roasted chiles, spices, ground cacao, and seeds. Different regions in Mexico have their own version, and moles can vary in color from dark red, to brown, black, green, and yellow. The most commonly known mole sauce is dark red in color, like the one featured here. The mole in this recipe is featured on roasted duck breasts, but you could use it in a number of ways: as a sauce for enchiladas (known as *enmoladas*), with eggs, or with pieces of chicken or beef. Mole's bold character would also make a striking complement to a delicate fillet of white flaky fish.

Yield: Approximately 5 cups

¼ cup lard, divided in thirds

2 ounces (approximately 6) dried pasilla/negro chiles, cored and seeded

1 ounce (approximately 2) dried ancho chiles, cored and seeded

1 ounce (approximately 6) dried New Mexico chiles, cored and seeded

1 small onion, sliced

1 clove garlic, sliced

¼ cup almonds, blanched and chopped

¼ cup raisins

1 tablespoon sesame seeds

¼ teaspoon star anise, ground

¼ teaspoon cloves, ground

1 small tomato, peeled, cored, seeded, and chopped (about ¼ cup)

2 ounces baking chocolate, 70–80% cacao, chopped

1 quart duck or chicken bone broth

2 tablespoons coconut (palm) sugar

2 teaspoons salt

1. Heat one-third of the lard in a large, heavy-bottomed pan (cast iron is ideal). Fry the chiles on all sides, turning them with tongs. Transfer to a pot with water, bring to a boil, and turn off the heat. Set them aside for a few minutes until the chiles soften.

2. While the chiles soak, use another one-third of the lard to sauté the onions over medium heat. When the onions turn translucent, add the garlic, almonds, raisins, sesame seeds, star anise, cloves, and tomato. Drain the chiles and add them to the mix. The mixture will be fragrant at this point. Allow all the flavors to merge over low heat. After a few minutes, add the chocolate, stirring the whole time until it melts. Remove from the heat immediately.

3. Transfer to a blender and add the bone broth. Blend until you have a smooth, thick sauce.

4. Warm the last third of the lard over medium heat and return the sauce to the pan. Be cautious—the sauce will splatter easily. After about 5 minutes, add the sugar and salt. Taste and adjust the seasoning to your liking.

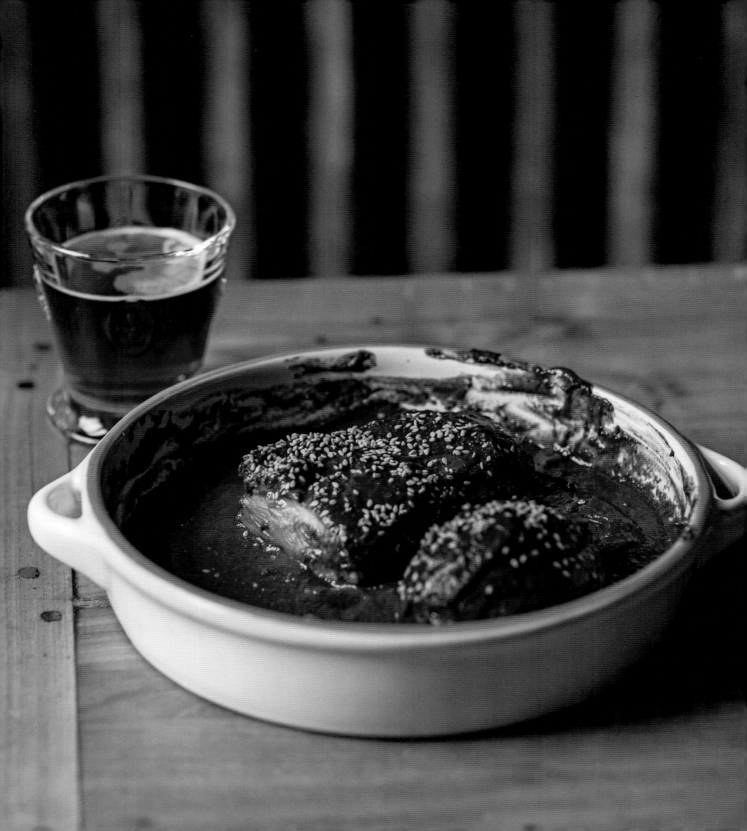

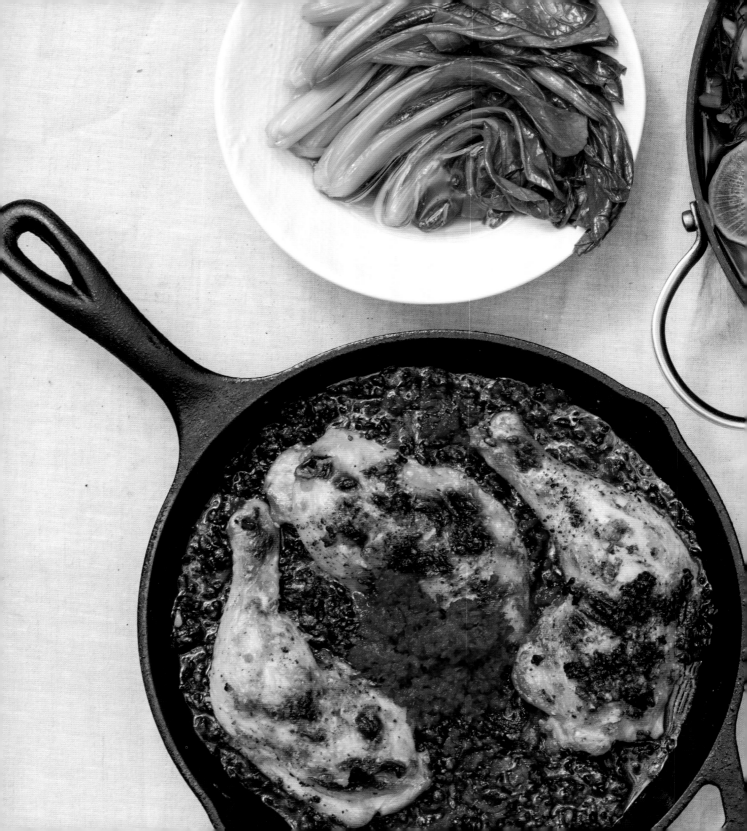

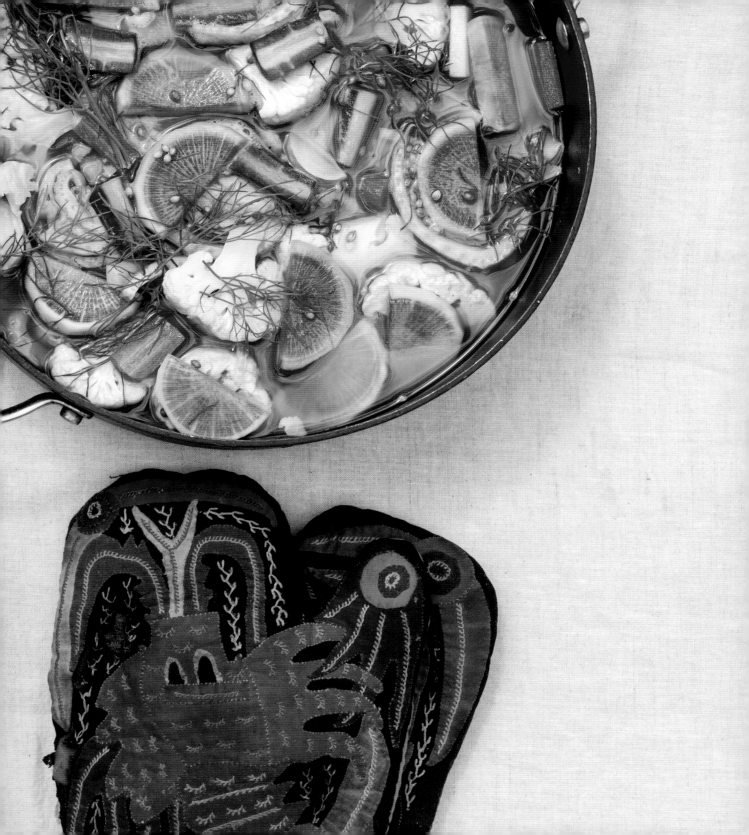

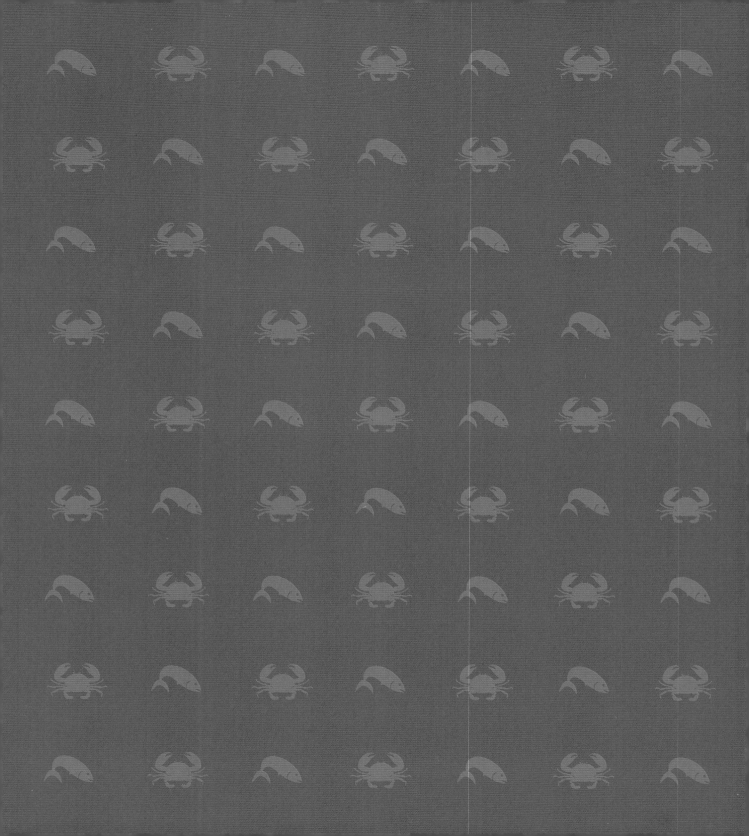

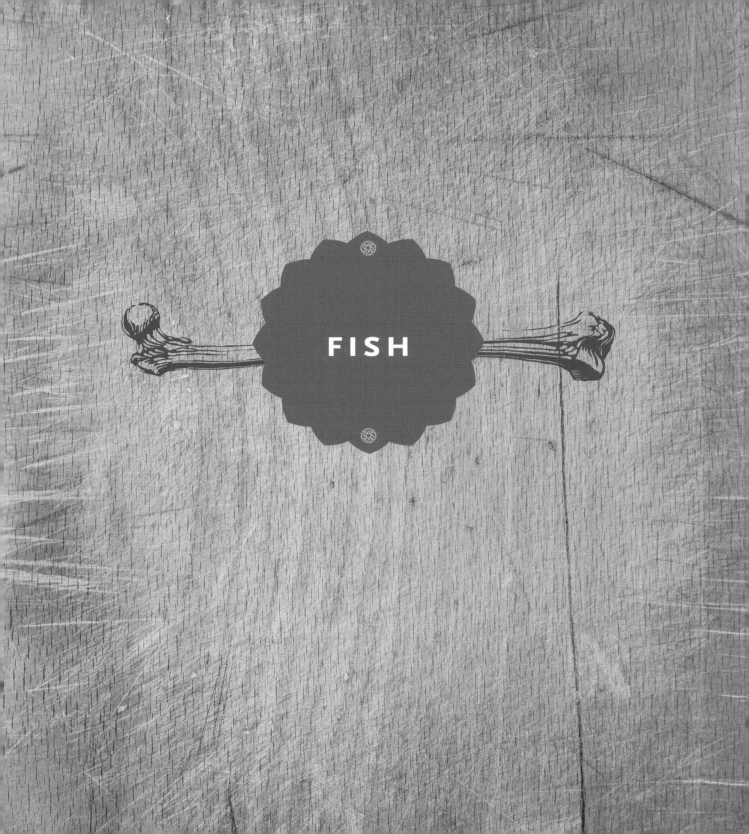

FISH

Seafood Miso Soup

THIS SOUP IS PREPARED SIMILARLY TO HOW YOU WOULD PREPARE TRADITIONAL JAPANESE FISH SOUPS served in hot pots. For this recipe, we used monkfish because its firm and creamy texture holds together well in soups. If you do not know monkish, it is often compared to lobster in both texture and flavor. Grouper, snapper, and halibut make good substitutes. Fish broth is the base for this soup, with added dried bonito (fish) flakes and kombu seaweed, both commonly used to flavor soup stocks in Japan. Bonito flakes impart a salty, slightly smoky flavor to the broth. Kombu provides an extra mineral boost and is used frequently in Chinese medicine to reduce phlegm and to treat some types of thyroid imbalances. Serve this soup with steamed rice, rice noodles, or buckwheat noodles.

Yield: 4 servings

1 3-inch piece kelp or kombu seaweed

6 cups fish bone broth

4 carrots, chopped

½ cup dried bonito flakes

1 leek, sliced

2 scallions, sliced

1 cup daikon radish, julienned

1 cup shiitake mushrooms, sliced

1 cup sliced pieces winter squash, such as acorn or butternut

1 tablespoon sake or white wine

1 tablespoon mirin

2 fillets monkfish (about 14 ounces), cubed

12 clams

2 tablespoons white miso

Gomashio (a Japanese condiment made of a mix of roasted sesame seeds and salt)

Ginger root, peeled and shredded

Pickled vegetables

1. In a large pot, soak the kelp or kombu seaweed in the fish broth for 30 minutes. Turn on the heat, and when the water begins to simmer and almost reaches a boil, remove the seaweed. Add the carrots and simmer for another 30 minutes. Add the bonito flakes and turn off the heat immediately. Cover and let it rest for 5 minutes. Strain the broth and discard the solids.

2. Bring the broth back to a simmer and add the leek, scallions, radish, mushrooms, and squash. Simmer for 15 minutes. Add the sake, mirin, fish, and clams. When the fish and the clams cook through (the clams should open up when ready), about 8–10 minutes, add the white miso, mix well, and turn off the heat.

3. Garnish with gomashio, ginger, and pickled vegetables, and serve over rice or noodles.

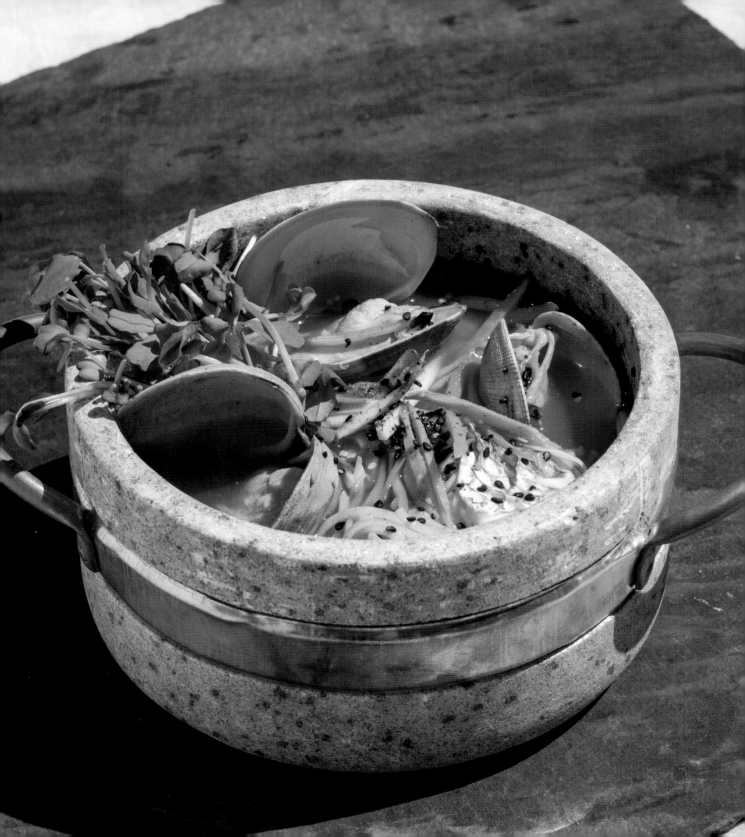

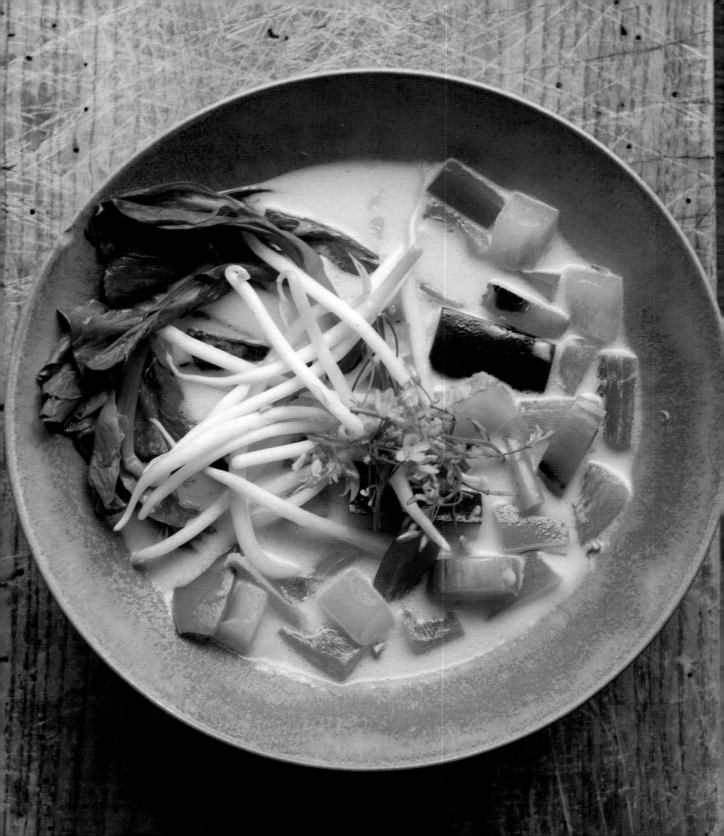

Yellow Thai Curry

WE LOVE THAI CURRIES, AND WE ESPECIALLY LOVE THE PROCESS OF MAKING THEM.
The scent of each ingredient as it comes into contact with the heat releases aromas
that are mouthwatering. We use fish broth here and recommend having it with chunks
of firm-flesh white fish. You can also use beef broth, and although this recipe calls
for vegetables only, it is also great with thinly sliced steak.

Yield: 4 servings

YELLOW CURRY CHILE PASTE

8 cloves garlic, unpeeled

10 bird chiles (dried Thai chiles),
or chiles de árbol

1 inch-long chunk ginger root,
unpeeled

4 shallots, unpeeled

1 teaspoon white peppercorns

1 teaspoon coriander seeds

1 teaspoon cumin seeds

1 teaspoon salt

1 tablespoon curry powder

1 teaspoon red miso

CURRY PASTE

1. Heat the oven to 375°F. Roast the garlic until soft, 10–12 minutes. Allow to cool, then peel.

2. In a cast-iron skillet, dry-roast the chiles over high heat until charred. Set the chiles aside and add the ginger and shallots, 15 minutes or so, turning them once during that time. Set the ginger and shallots aside.

3. Add the white peppercorns to the skillet and dry-roast for a few minutes or until fragrant. Set aside. Repeat the dry-roasting process with the coriander seeds and then the cumin seeds.

4. Discard the stems from the chiles and mince. Peel the ginger and shallots and mince. Set aside.

5. Use a mortar to pound the salt and garlic to form a paste. One ingredient at a time, add the chiles, ginger, shallots, peppercorn, coriander, cumin, curry powder, and miso, making sure each ingredient is fully incorporated before adding the next. The paste will keep in an airtight container, refrigerated, for up to a month.

(Continued)

CURRY BROTH

CURRY BROTH

1½ cups full fat coconut milk

1½ cups fish or beef bone broth

1 teaspoon salt

2 tablespoons fish sauce or soy sauce

2 teaspoons coconut sugar

1 stalk lemongrass, tough outer layers removed, chopped and pounded

6–7 kaffir lime leaves, crushed (you may use dried kaffir leaves), or the grated zest of 1 lime

4 cups mixed seasonal vegetables, chopped into bite-size pieces

GARNISH

Fresh cilantro, mint, and/or basil leaves, roughly chopped

1. Combine the coconut milk and chile paste. If you prefer a less spicy curry, don't add all of the paste and save for another use.

2. In a saucepan over medium heat, warm the coconut-chile mixture, stirring frequently. Add the bone broth and stir to mix.

3. When the mixture reaches a simmer, add the salt, fish sauce, coconut sugar, lemongrass, and lime leaves. Reduce the heat to medium-low and simmer for 15–20 minutes. (If making the curry broth ahead, let cool completely at this point and refrigerate. It will keep overnight.)

4. Add the vegetables to the simmering broth. Remember to start with the densest vegetables, such as root vegetables, first. When they soften, add the more tender and quicker-cooking vegetables, like broccoli, cauliflower, and peas.

5. Once the vegetables are cooked through, serve immediately. Garnish with chopped fresh cilantro, mint, and/or basil.

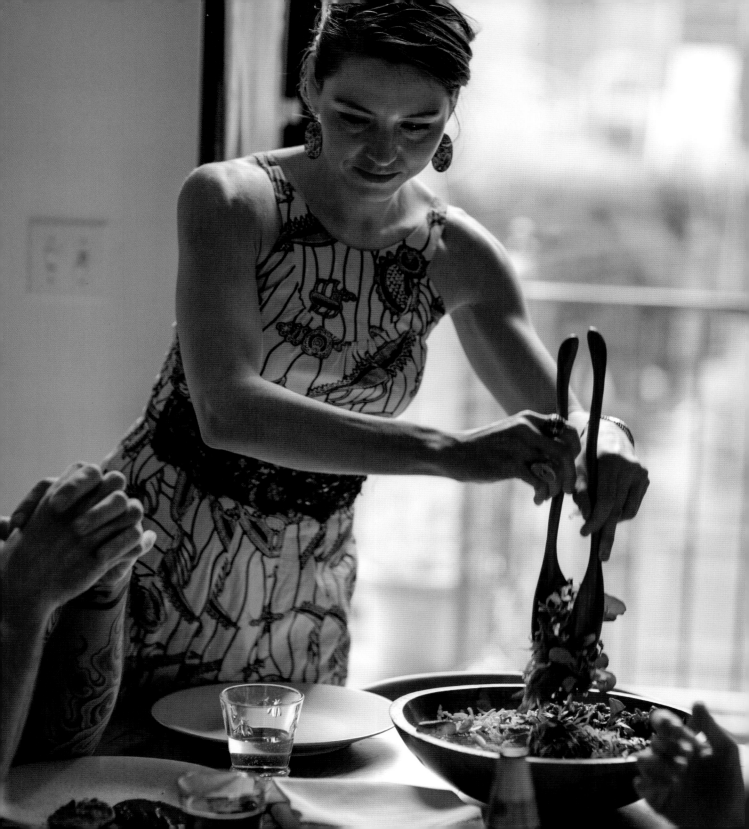

Mussels in Broth
with Tomato, Fennel, and Saffron

MUSSELS ARE A PERFECT VEHICLE FOR BRIGHT AND FLAVORFUL BROTHS, LIKE THE ONE IN THIS RECIPE, which pays homage to a classic bouillabaisse. Pernod, saffron, fennel, cured salami, and mussels come together to transport you to the south of France through the portal of your palate. This recipe makes a beautiful family-style meal, and we love serving it for summer dinners on our roof deck alongside a large salad of farmers market greens, our favorite crusty bread, and a great bottle (or two!) of white or rosé.

Yield: 4 servings as a main dish, more if using as an appetizer

2 tablespoons extra virgin olive oil

4 ounces hard, dry fennel salami, diced

1 small bulb fennel, thinly sliced (about 1 cup)

1 small onion, thinly sliced (about 1 cup)

4 medium cloves garlic, thinly sliced

Kosher salt and freshly ground black pepper

Pinch saffron

Pinch red pepper flakes

¼ cup pastis or Pernod

1 piece orange zest

½ cup crushed tomatoes

3–4 cups fish bone broth

2 pounds mussels

3 tablespoons minced fresh parsley leaves

1 tablespoon butter

1 tablespoon fresh lemon juice

1 loaf rustic sourdough bread

1. Heat the oil in a large saucepan over high heat until shimmering. Add the salami and cook, stirring, for 30 seconds. Add the fennel, onion, and garlic. Reduce the heat to medium, season with salt and pepper, and cook, stirring, until the vegetables are softened, about 5 minutes.

2. Add the saffron and pepper flakes and cook until fragrant, about 30 seconds. Add the pastis, orange zest, and tomatoes. Add the broth, increase the heat to high, and bring to a boil.

3. Add the mussels, cover, and cook, shaking the pan constantly and stirring every 30 seconds.

2. As soon as all the mussels are open, reduce heat to a simmer and transfer mussels to a bowl using tongs. Place the pan lid over the bowl to keep the mussels warm. Remove the broth from the heat and whisk in the parsley, butter, and lemon juice. Return the mussels to the pot, stir to combine, then transfer to a large serving bowl. Serve immediately with broiled bread.

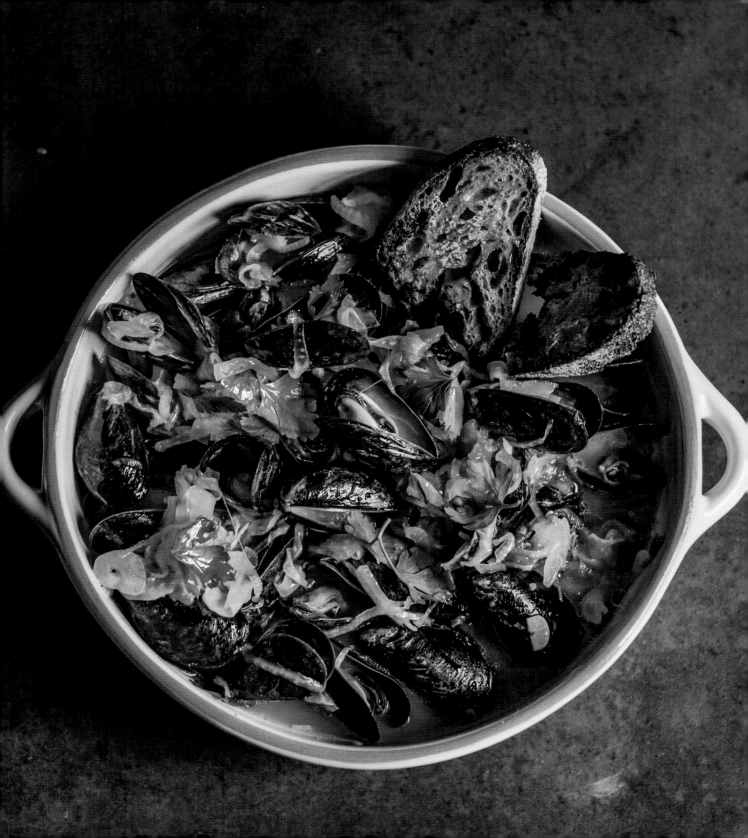

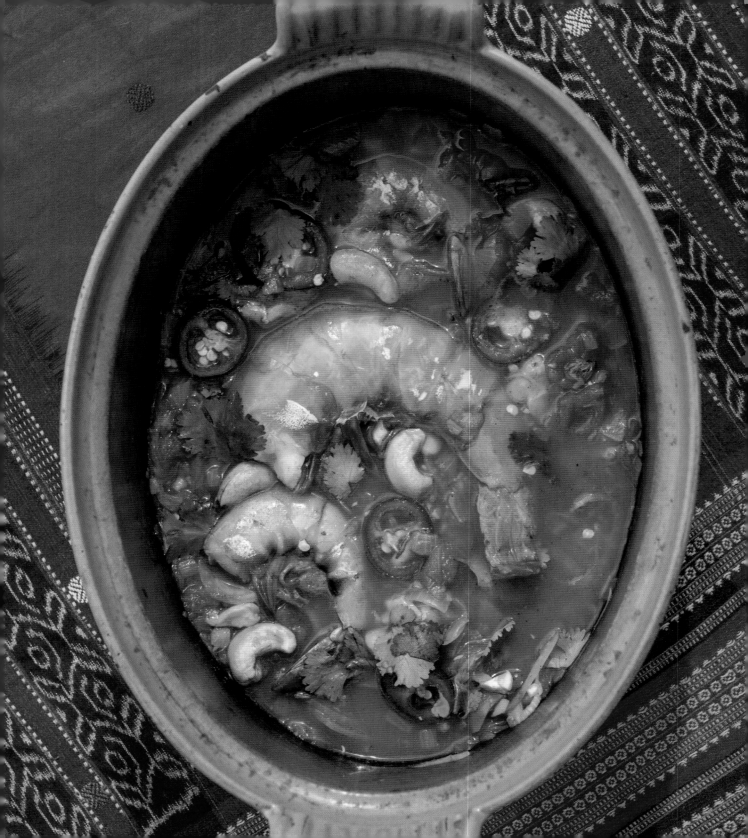

Spicy Prawn Stew

THIS RECIPE IS OUR TRIBUTE TO A CREAMY COCONUT PRAWN DISH THAT IS TRADITIONAL TO Bengal. We substitute the use of coconut milk with tomatoes and fennel for a lighter dish that makes a fantastic summer meal. The sauce may be prepared a day in advance. Just bring to a quick boil, reduce the heat immediately, and add the prawns when you're ready to serve.

Yield: 4 servings

1 tablespoon olive oil

1 cup onions, chopped (about 1 onion)

1 teaspoon coriander seeds, toasted and ground

¼ teaspoon ground turmeric

1 clove garlic, minced

1 tablespoon ginger root, finely chopped (about 1 thumb-sized piece)

1 cup tomatoes, peeled, and diced (about 3 small–medium size)

1 cup fennel, sliced (about 1 small bulb)

2 cups fish bone broth

1½ pounds prawns (or about 4 prawns per person)

1 jalapeño or serrano pepper, thinly sliced (optional)

1 small handful fresh cilantro, chopped

¼ cup dry-roasted cashews

1. Warm the olive oil in a medium cast-iron pan. Add the onions and cook over medium-low heat until soft, about 8 minutes.

2. Add the coriander and turmeric and mix well. When fragrant, about 1 minute, add the garlic, ginger, tomatoes, and fennel. Cook for 10 minutes, stirring occasionally.

3. Add the bone broth and bring to a boil. Reduce the heat immediately and allow the sauce to simmer over low heat for another 10 minutes. Add the prawns, cover the pan, and cook about 5–7 minutes. Be sure to not overcook the prawns, or they will become very rubbery.

4. Garnish with the pepper, cilantro, and cashews and serve immediately.

THE DIFFERENCE BETWEEN PRAWNS AND SHRIMP

Most people use the terms *shrimp* and *prawns* interchangeably. They look very similar, but they are not the same . Prawns tend to be a little larger in size and have longer legs. They taste similar and can be used interchangeably in recipes. Ideally, purchase from local fishmongers whom you trust and who can give you information on the origin of their seafood. Northern shrimp and spot prawns are safer choices. See our Resources guide for a seafood company that we trust.

Malaysian Laksa

THIS MALAYSIAN CURRY BOASTS LAYERS OF FLAVOR AND TEXTURE,
at once festive and comforting. The recipe was inspired by Taylor's dear childhood friend and real
food aficionado, Marie Cudennec. Her original recipe calls for a prawn/chicken broth
and fresh prawns in the final dish. We've substituted fish broth and fish, as much of our family
has a shellfish allergy (at home we also leave out the dried shrimp), and it drastically reduces
the prep time! If using fish, a soft and flaky white fish works best. Choose a variety that is
as local to you as possible.

**You can double the recipe for the curry paste here and have it on hand for later in the week, perhaps
for a quick dinner of curried vegetables and rice, as a spread on eggs, or to flavor your morning broth.
The sambal recipe also has a generous yield and is a great addition to the condiments in your fridge.

Yield: 4 servings

4 tablespoons dried shrimp

10 red Thai chiles

3 teaspoons galangal (use ginger if you can't get galangal)

6 macadamia nuts

3 teaspoons grated fresh turmeric root

3 garlic cloves

8 small shallots

3 drops lemongrass essential oil

1 tablespoon coconut oil

4 cups fish bone broth

Sea salt, to taste

Coconut sugar, to taste

1 cup organic rice noodles, uncooked

⅓ cup organic full-fat coconut milk

1 pound flaky white fish

1. Blend the shrimp, chiles, galangal, nuts, turmeric, garlic, shallots, and lemongrass oil in a blender to make a curry paste.

2. Heat the coconut oil in a heavy-bottomed pot (we like cast iron or ceramic), add the fresh curry paste, and cook until fragrant.

3. Add the broth directly into the pot with the cooked curry paste. Mix thoroughly.

4. Add sea salt and coconut sugar to taste and allow the broth to simmer over medium heat for 10–15 minutes. Meanwhile, blanch the noodles in a separate pot of boiling water, strain, and set aside for serving.

5. Stir the coconut milk into the curry. Allow the broth to come to a boil, then add the fish. Reduce to a simmer and flake the fish apart as it cooks. Remove from the heat as soon as the fish is cooked—the flaky, buttery texture can quickly turn chewy if overcooked.

(Continued)

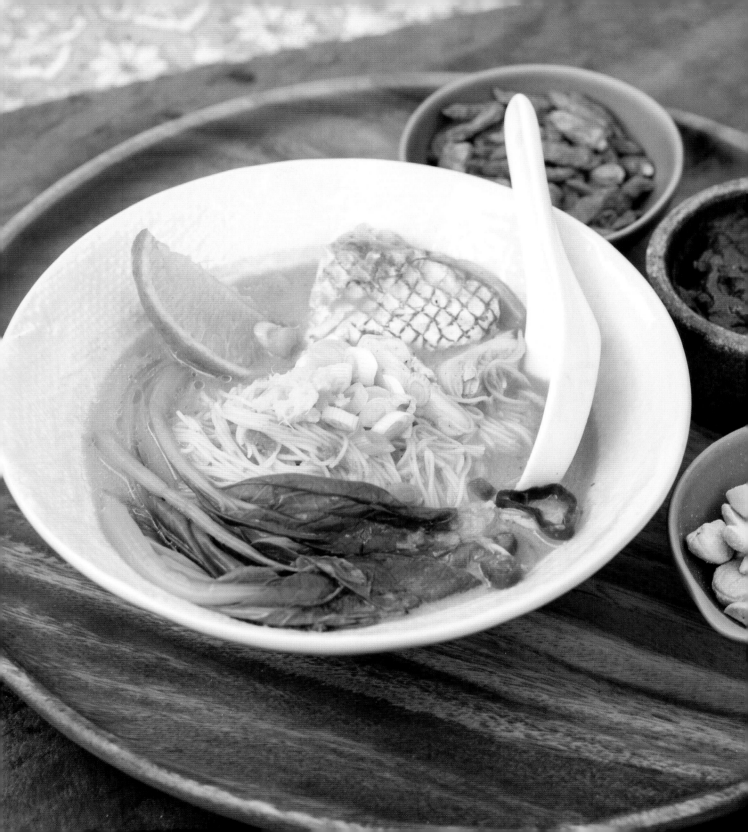

Sambal (recipe below)

Fresh cilantro or mint

Mung bean sprouts

Soft-boiled egg

A few thin slices of organic cucumber

Fresh lime wedges

15 dried red Thai chiles, soaked and seeds removed

3 cloves garlic, peeled

1 tablespoon coconut milk

1 teaspoon tamarind paste

1 shallot, finely sliced

1 tablespoon anchovies

⅓ cup water

Sea salt, to taste

Unrefined sugar, to taste

Coconut oil for frying

6. To serve, divide the cooked noodles into bowls, add curried broth, and your preferred garnishes. We love a mix of sprouts, green herbs, crunchy cucumber, and soft-boiled egg to provide a pop of color and texture. Serve with sambal.

SAMBAL

Yield: roughly ⅔ cup

1. Place the chiles, garlic, coconut milk, tamarind paste, shallot, anchovies, water, salt, and sugar in a blender and blend to form a smooth paste.

2. Heat a small knob of coconut oil in a frying pan. Transfer the mixture into the hot oil and cook over medium-low heat for 5–10 minutes, until the color deepens. Remove from the pan and set aside for later. (This can be prepared in advance and stored in a jar in the refrigerator for 2 weeks.)

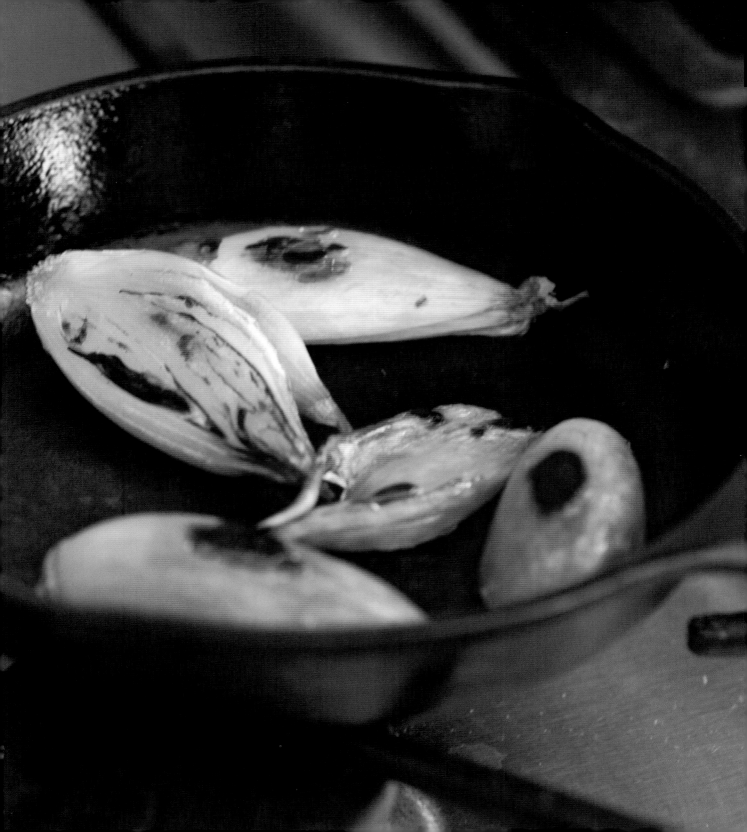

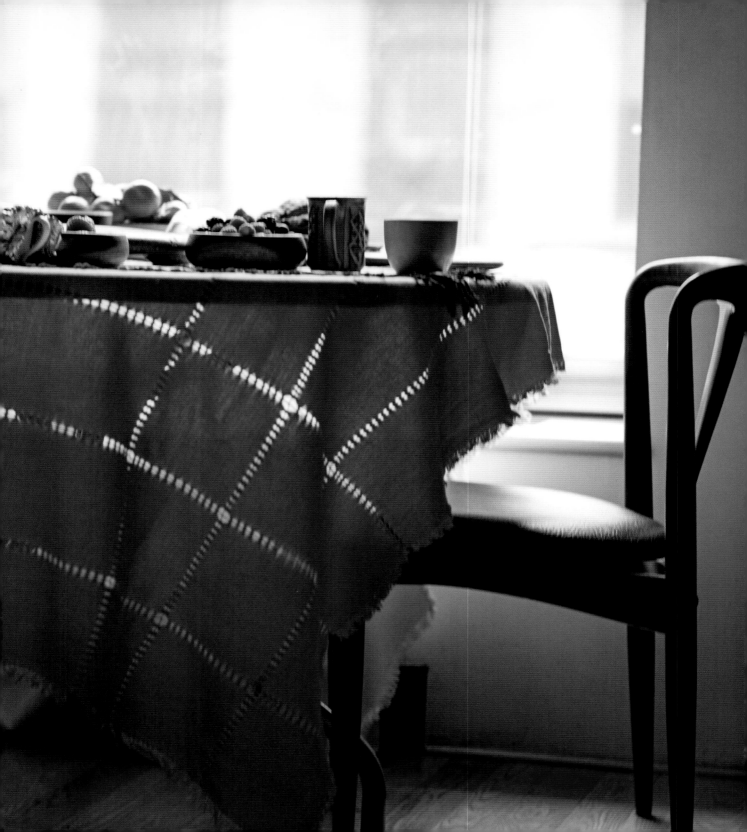

"Savoring bone broth is an opportunity to connect to the wisdom of our elders; it has always been a sacred and primal food, nourishing us through challenging and redefining moments. Pregnancy and childbirth, the most primitive experiences a woman will have in our modern time, require the building and healing elements that good broth can provide."

—*Emily Brown,*
**FERTILITY FOODS CHEF BASED IN NYC,
AND FOUNDER OF FERTILE GROUND KITCHEN**

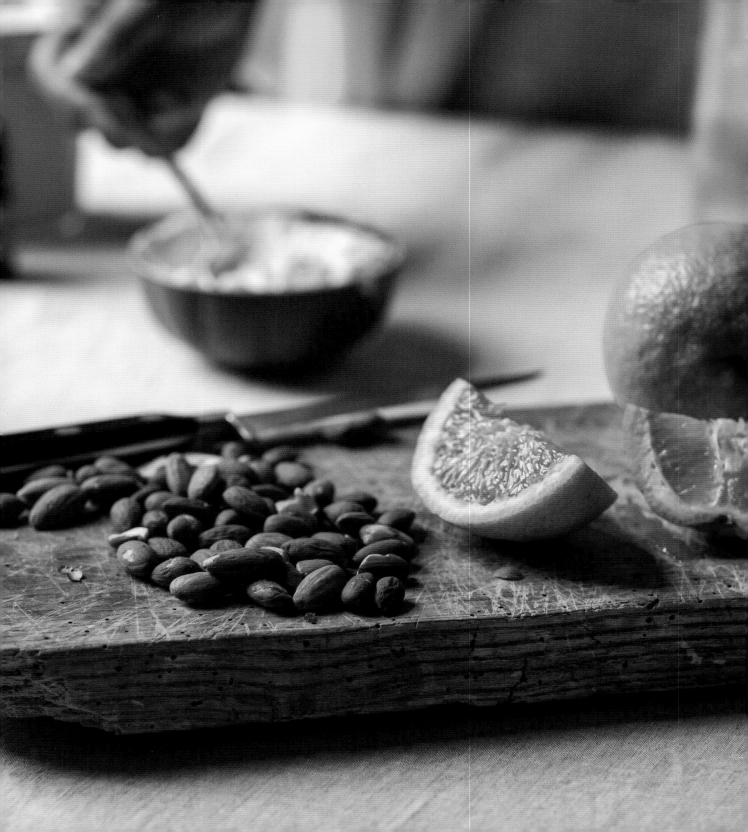

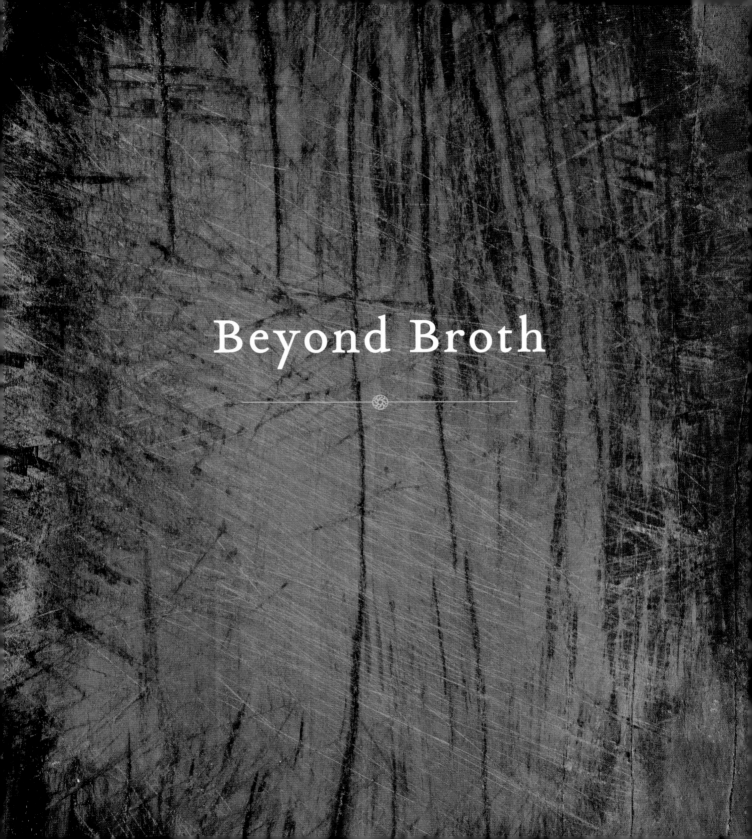

Beyond Broth

I N THIS SECTION, WE INVITE YOU TO EXPLORE bone broth as inspiration for more sustainable and creative living. While we began consuming broth years ago for its obvious health benefits, what has arisen over time is an awareness of the idea of nose-to-tail eating and living, a remembrance of the resourcefulness and creativity of our ancestors. Not only does consuming the whole animal provide a full spectrum of nutrition, but there is utility in the leftovers, too. Traditionally the hides were set aside for clothing and shelter, the hooves for making glue, and the fat used for making candles and soap. The nose-to-tail lifestyle is a more conscientious choice for the environment by using more and wasting less, and consuming and utilizing the whole animal supports the whole human inside and out.

One of our most exciting projects lately has been collaborating with our dear friend and soap maker Erica Robinson on a line of soaps and balms made from our own tallow. Tallow, the rendered fat from cattle, makes a fantastically hydrating and lathery soap; it also makes our favorite all-natural multipurpose balm, which is extra nourishing without leaving a greasy residue.

In the following pages you'll find recipes for using clean tallow to make your own luxurious soaps and silky skin balms. These recipes are incredibly simple and require little time to make so you can really have fun taking time experimenting with your own favorite scents and essential oils. We love gifting these goodies, and our friends always love receiving custom beauty products from honest ingredients.

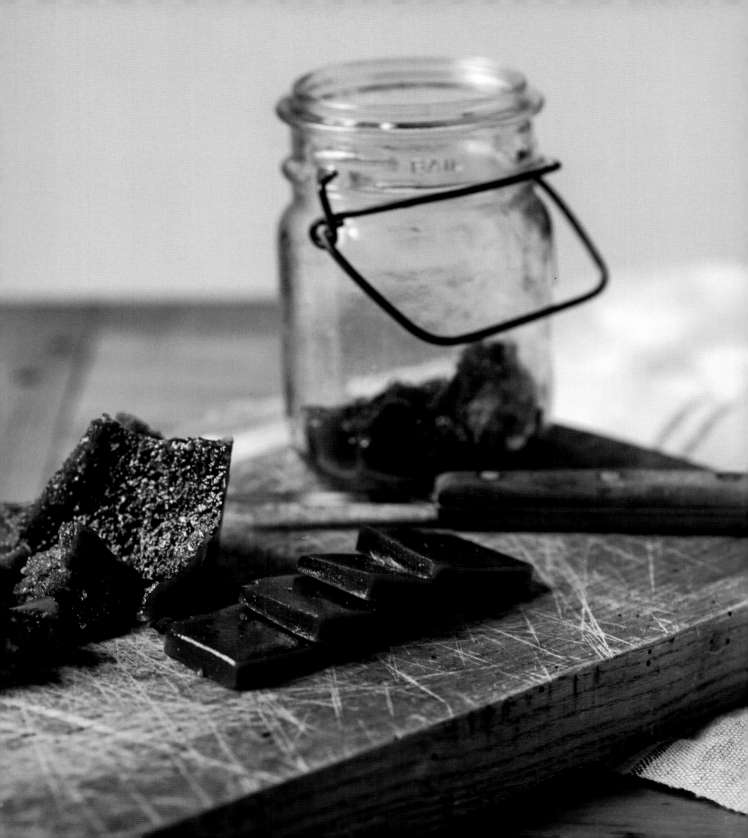

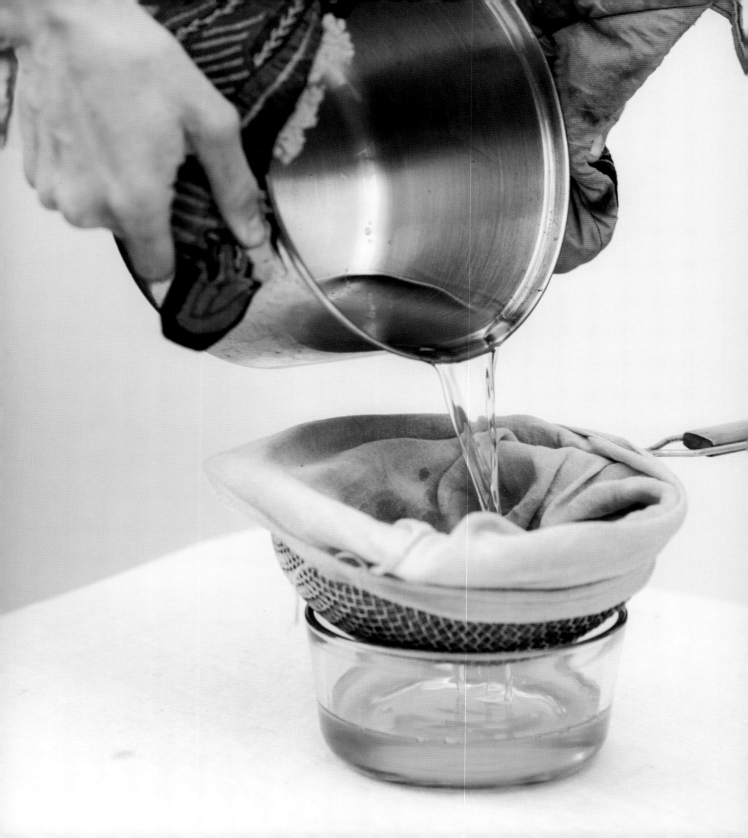

Rendering Tallow

BUTCHERS END UP WITH AN ABUNDANCE OF FAT scraps at the end of the day, which we use to produce tallow. Tallow is the fat rendered from beef. It has 50–55 percent saturated fat and 40 percent monounsaturated fat content; it is very stable and great for frying. Ask your local butcher to save you some fat scraps. Fat scraps are inexpensive, as they often go to waste. You may follow the same method of rendering fat for any other animal fat. We often make lard (pig fat), as it also performs well for cooking at higher temperatures.

There are a few ways to render tallow. One of them is by making beef bone broth. The fat that congeals at the top of the broth during the cooling process may be lifted from the broth. That tallow can be used as a cooking fat. If you wish to store tallow rendered in this way, you must remove all meat solids and broth liquid. Otherwise, the tallow will go bad quickly. To do this, remove the congealed fat from the top of the cooled broth and melt the fat over low heat. Allow the liquid to cool for 10 minutes, then strain it through a fine sieve or cheesecloth while it is still liquid. Store in a tightly sealed glass container in the refrigerator for up to 1 year.

We use the method above for use in cooking, mainly because the broth that we make includes onions, garlic, and other aromatics that will infuse the fat and add more flavor to the foods cooked with it. If you wish to have pure unflavored tallow, prepare plain bone broth using only the bones and water or follow the recipe provided on the next page. The quality of the tallow rendered in this recipe is good for use in non-food preparations that require unflavored tallow, as is the case in our soap and balm recipes.

Tallow

1 pound fat, chopped

1. Preheat the oven to 220°F. Place the chopped fat in the steamer basket of a stainless steel steamer pot. Place the pot in the oven and bake for 4 hours or until all the fat has dripped from the steamer basket into the steamer pot. Use a wooden spoon to press the fat down a few times in the oven during the rendering time, until all the fat has dripped into the pot and you are left with only crispy chips of fat in the steamer basket. Remove the pot from the oven and discard the chips.

2. Line a mixing bowl with a few layers of cheesecloth. Pour the fat from the pot through the cheesecloth. Discard any solids strained by the cheesecloth. The strained fat is your tallow, which at this point will be a golden liquid. Transfer to a clean glass jar and allow it to cool. As it cools, it will turn into a white, creamy paste. Seal the jar tightly, label and date it, and store in the refrigerator for up to 1 year, or in the freezer for even longer storage.

A NOTE ON FATS

Fat is a necessary, nourishing food. Thankfully, the fat-free paradigm of the past few decades is shifting as modern research clarifies that not all fat is bad. Rather, particular types of chemically altered fats, as well as "good" fats that have gone rancid from improper storage or cooking, are toxic to our systems. The fact is, the body needs both saturated and unsaturated fats for well-being. Fats make up cell walls, which mediate the passage of vital or harmful substances in and out.

Saturated fats are found primarily in animal foods but also in coconut and palm oils. Real saturated fats, such as butter, ghee, tallow, and coconut oil, are heat stable. In other words, these fats can maintain their integrity at higher temperatures and are not readily altered or oxidized during cooking. Saturated fats in foods like red meat and full-fat dairy are useful for maintaining a healthy digestive tract and helping bones build calcium. They also aid in the synthesis of essential fatty acids and fat-soluble vitamins.

Unsaturated fats are sourced primarily from plant foods and fish and are divided into two categories: monounsaturated and polyunsaturated. Foods rich in monounsaturated fats include avocados, almonds, macadamia nuts, olives, and their oils. Foods rich in polyunsaturated fats include grain products, peanuts, and fish oils.

Plant-based oils are best unrefined and cold-pressed. With the exception of coconut oil, they are best used for finishing dishes, as salad dressings, or for dips. Because unsaturated fats are less stable, they go rancid more readily. If these oils are stored for extended periods in a hot cabinet over the stove and/or used for high-heat frying, they can form harmful free radicals that cause inflammation in the body.

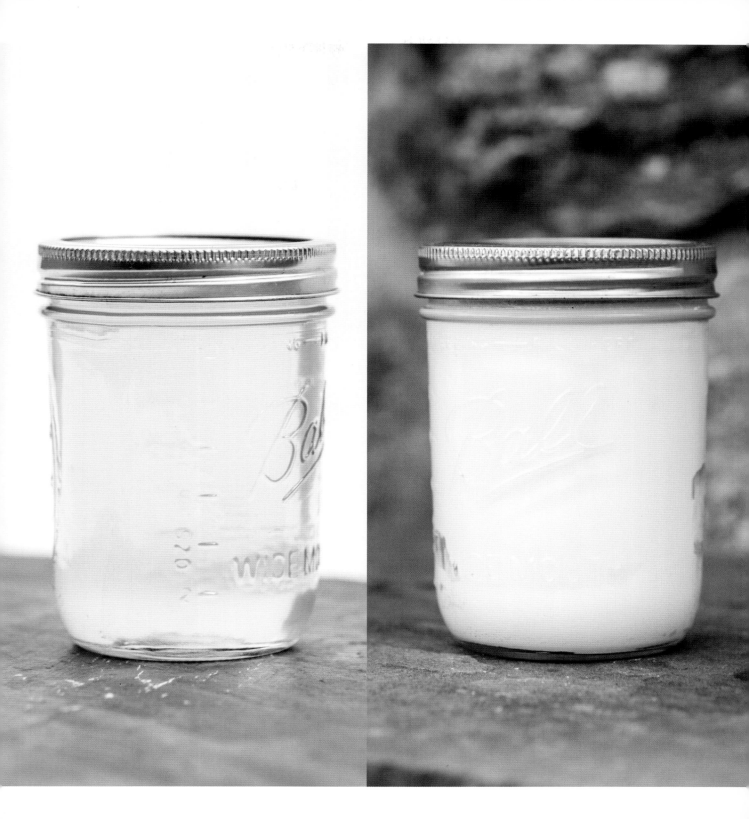

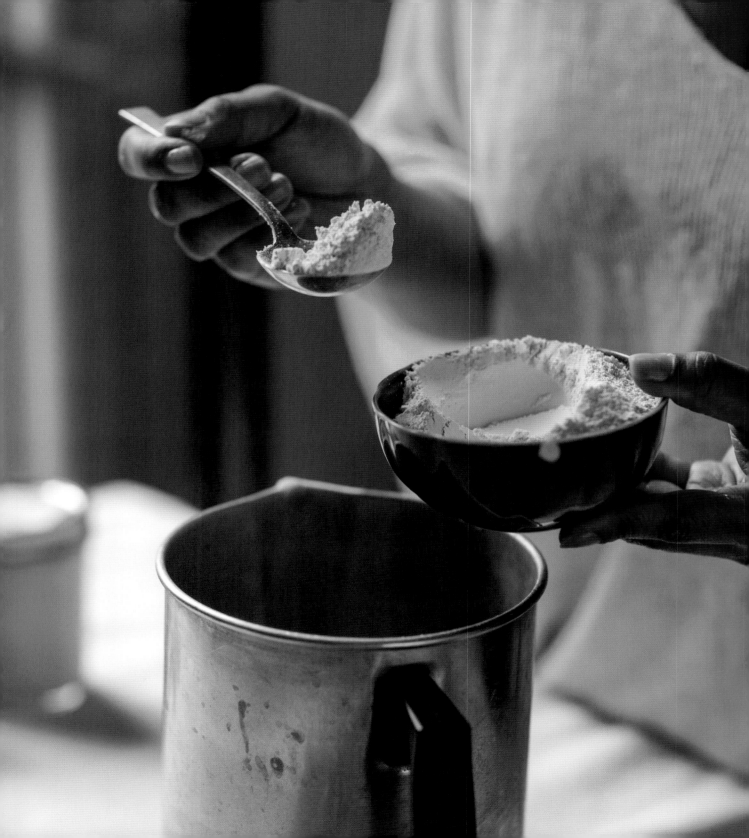

Tallow Soaps

THERE ARE TWO WAYS TO USE TALLOW IN SOAP making. One way is to saponify (that is, combine with alkali to form soap) the tallow itself. This method involves heating a precise amount of tallow (or other fat, such as olive or palm oil) to a specific temperature, combining it with a precise amount of lye (a strong alkaline liquor rich in potassium carbonate leached from wood ashes), then mixing for an extended time until the lye is fully incorporated. The resulting mixture is poured into molds and must be cured for many weeks. This is a long and tricky process, because lye is a caustic material and the ingredient measurements must be precise to ensure that no lye remains in the finished soap. The other method is to use tallow as a moisturizing additive to an already saponified vegetable soap base.

Both methods can work well; however, when it comes to using tallow, we prefer using it as an additive to a saponified olive oil base because we find the soap to be a better cleanser and it lathers up more while retaining the conditioning quality of the tallow. It also allows the essence of the fragrances of essential oils or absolutes to shine through with a bit more clarity as opposed to the other method, in which the tallow can overpower an essence. A little bit of tallow goes a long way in this recipe.

Tallow Soap

TO MOLD YOUR SOAP, YOU MAY USE A MILK CARTON OR OTHER RECTANGULAR SHAPE
and then cut the cooled soap into bars, or use molds with specific cavities and shapes.
Larger molds will yield fewer bars of soap.

Yield: 5 4-ounce bars

1 pound saponified olive or palm oil base (preferably organic)

1 ounce unrefined, filtered yellow beeswax

2 teaspoons tallow

1 tablespoon raw honey

1 tablespoon finely ground clay (bentonite, sea clay, pink clay)

1–3 teaspoons essential oil (this can be a single oil or a blend, but be sure not to use more than 3 teaspoons total or the soap may become too oily)

1. Heat 1 quart water in the bottom portion of a 2 quart double boiler. Cut the soap base into smaller chunks and place in the top pot. Add the beeswax and stir as it begins to melt together. Add the tallow and honey and stir until well blended.

2. Sift the clay slowly through a strainer to avoid chunks and blend until incorporated. Turn off the heat.

2. Add the essential oil and stir slowly until well blended. Carefully pour the mixture into the molds. Let sit for a few hours until completely hard. Depending on your climate, placing the filled molds in the refrigerator will help with the hardening process and make the soap easier to pop out.

3. You may wrap the soap in butcher paper or place it in a box or cellophane bag for storage.

4. Enjoy your bubbly, moisturizing bar of soap!

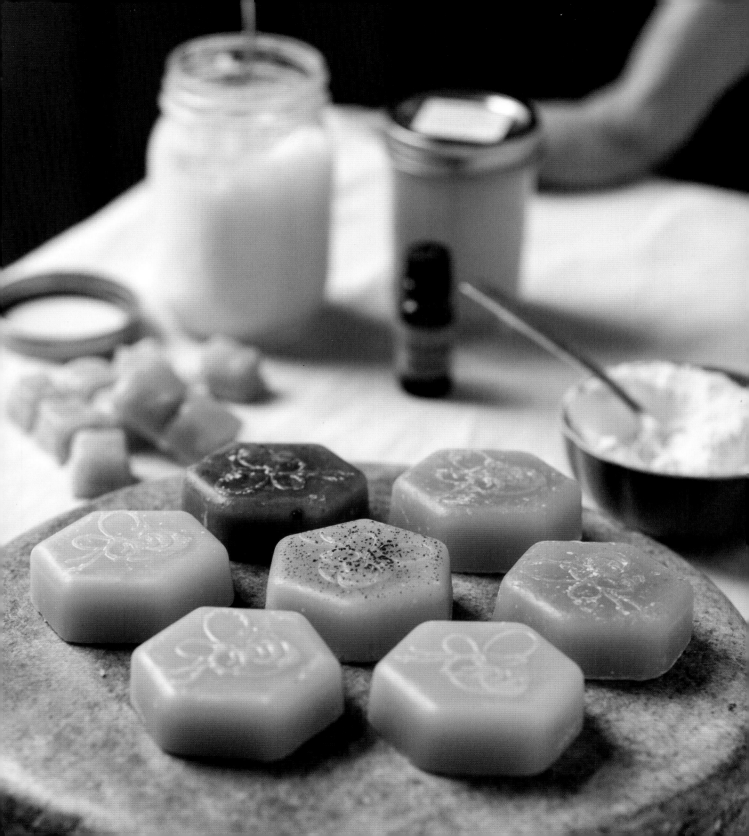

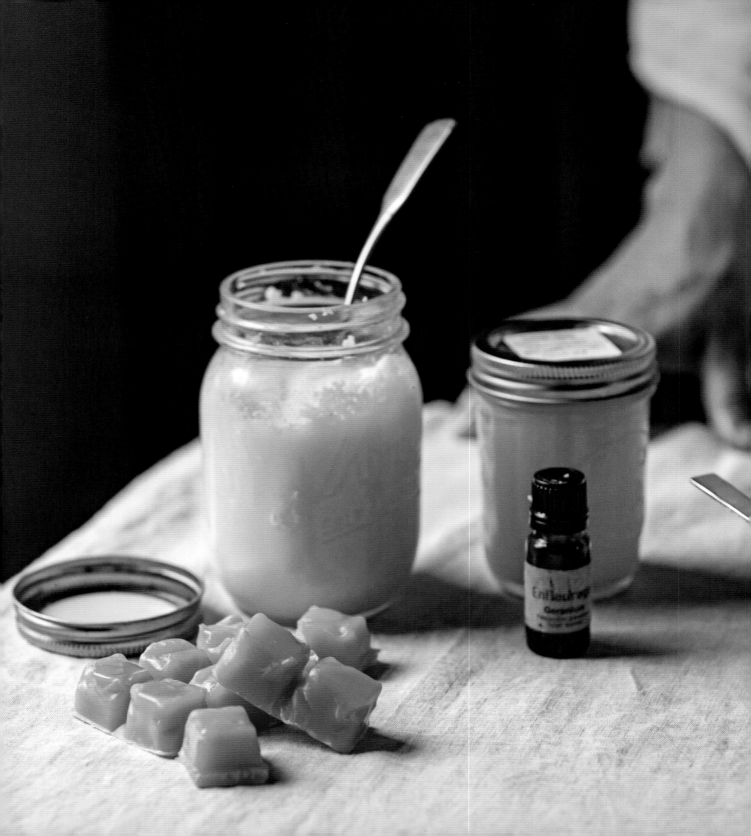

Tallow Lip Balm

TALLOW IS AN EXCELLENT MOISTURIZING CONDITIONER FOR SKIN AND LIPS.
In fact, some people who are allergic to commercial beauty products or have eczema can use tallow balms with ease. Below is an easy recipe to make a natural and nourishing lip balm.

Yield: Approximately 1½ ounces (6 small tubes or 3 small tins)

2 tablespoons jojoba oil

¾ teaspoon beef tallow

1–1¼ teaspoons grated, filtered yellow beeswax

10–15 drops essential oil of choice

Empty tins or tubes for storing lip balm

1. Combine the jojoba oil, tallow, and beeswax (use 1 teaspoon if putting your balm in a tin, or 1¼ teaspoons if putting your balm in a tube) in a small saucepan and heat on medium low until the tallow and beeswax are melted into the jojoba oil.

2. Add the essential oil of choice.

3. Pour your balm into your tins or tubes, cover, and wait for the balm to harden.

4. Enjoy your lip balm!

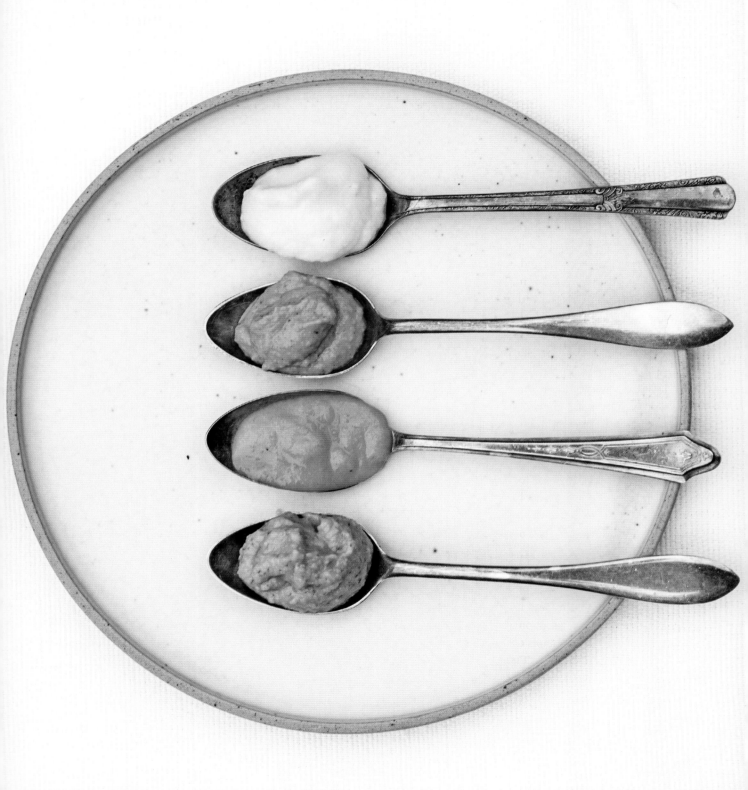

Bone Broth for Babies

IN A STUDY BY AGOSTINI ET AL PUBLISHED IN THE *Journal of the American College of Nutrition* in 2000 comparing the free amino acid profile of breast milk to that of various infant formulas, it was found that breast milk is rich in glutamic acid and glutamine. These amino acids are responsible for imparting the umami taste to foods. Umami is one of the five basic tastes—often described as the savory taste that is pleasant to most people. It may also be described as a "meaty" or "brothy" taste, and it is said to have an important role in making food taste delicious.

Our first contact with the umami flavor is through breast milk. In fact, the study found that breast milk and broth samples have a similar glutamate content. It is no wonder that babies naturally like bone broth! We have yet to meet a baby who doesn't. Most importantly, bone broth is a great first food for babies because of its easy digestibility and because it helps prepare babies' delicate GI tracts to receive new foods.

When we began our babies on solids, we did lots of research as to what to introduce, how frequently, and so on. One of the most important discoveries we made is that babies are not fully equipped with the enzymes necessary to process grains and most carbohydrates until age one, with the exception of mashed banana because the fruit itself contains the enzyme amylase, which babies need to digest it. The common practice of beginning babies on fortified cereals may be the culprit in developing grain allergies later down the line.

Babies' immature digestive systems are best equipped to digest fats and proteins early on (the basic composition of breast milk), making nutrient-dense foods, primarily animal foods, ideal. Ideal first foods include iron-rich liver (which replenishes babies' own stores of iron, which start to deplete around six months), yolks from pastured eggs (abundant with omega-3s, choline, and cholesterol, necessary for mental development), cod liver oil, and fish roe (with valuable vitamins A, D, and K, iodine, and DHA). Fruits and vegetables are best introduced later, between six and eight months, and mixed with plenty of fat to aid digestion.

When first beginning baby on solids, as a rule of thumb, introduce one food at a time to rule out any allergies. You can also test a baby's sensitivity to a new food by placing the food on the skin of his wrist before bed and watching for a reaction, such as itching or rash. Don't write off a new food completely if your baby reacts the first time it's introduced. Often you can try the same food a few weeks later and find your baby has no reaction.

Once a new food has the green light, feel free to combine multiple flavors. Additionally, don't be shy of adding "adult" flavors to your baby's food! Introducing strong flavors like garlic, onions, ginger, cod liver oil, Brussels sprouts, and so on early on tends to result in a toddler with a broader palate. Starting your baby on just sweet and starchy foods can make for fussy eaters later on.

When making baby foods at home, we use a basic recipe of broth-simmered vegetables or fruit mixed with a little cream or coconut oil. Often we add egg yolks or bone marrow to make a custard or include cod liver oil or small amounts of organ meats for superior nutrition. Following are basic guidelines for preparation and just a few suggested ingredient pairings.

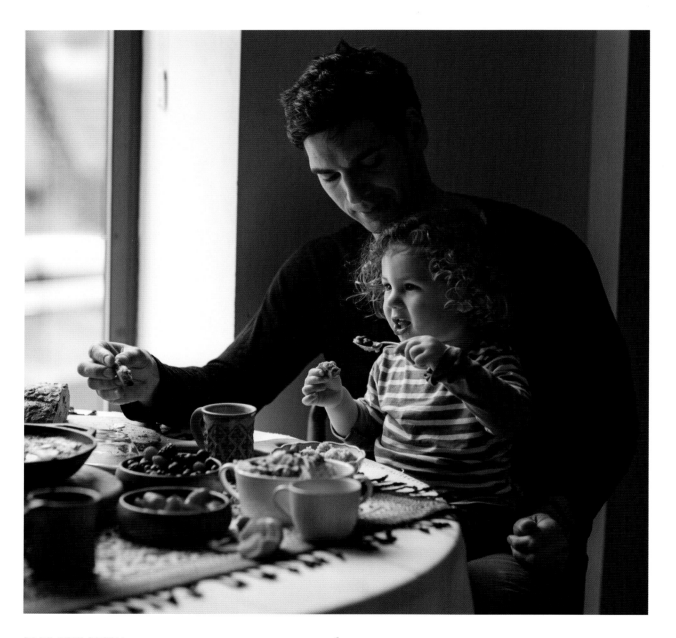

Baby Food Basic Instructions

CHERRY, APPLE, AND PARSNIP

1 organic apple, cubed

1–2 organic parsnip roots, depending on size, cubed

2 tablespoons organic unsweetened dried cherries, or ⅓ cup fresh

1 tablespoon coconut oil

BROCCOLI, SWEET PEA, AND MINT

1 cup organic broccoli florets

¾ cup organic sweet peas

5 organic fresh mint leaves (add only when blending; do not cook)

1 tablespoon grass-fed butter

BANANA AND PUMPKIN CUSTARD

2 organic bananas

1 cup cubed organic pumpkin or winter squash

2 soft egg yolks

CAULIFLOWER AND CELERIAC CUSTARD

1 cup cubed organic celeriac

1 cup organic cauliflower florets

¼ cup fresh (preferably raw) cream

3 tablespoons marrow

1. Chop whole fruit or vegetables into small chunks and place in small pot with enough broth to cover. Bring to a boil and immediately reduce to a simmer. Allow to cook until the fruit and vegetables are soft but still maintain their vibrant color.

2. Remove from the heat and allow to cool for 5–10 minutes.

3. Pour into a food processor or blender along with raw coconut oil or grass-fed butter. Pulse to the desired chunkiness or smoothness.

4. Stir in a soft-boiled egg yolk or cooked marrow.

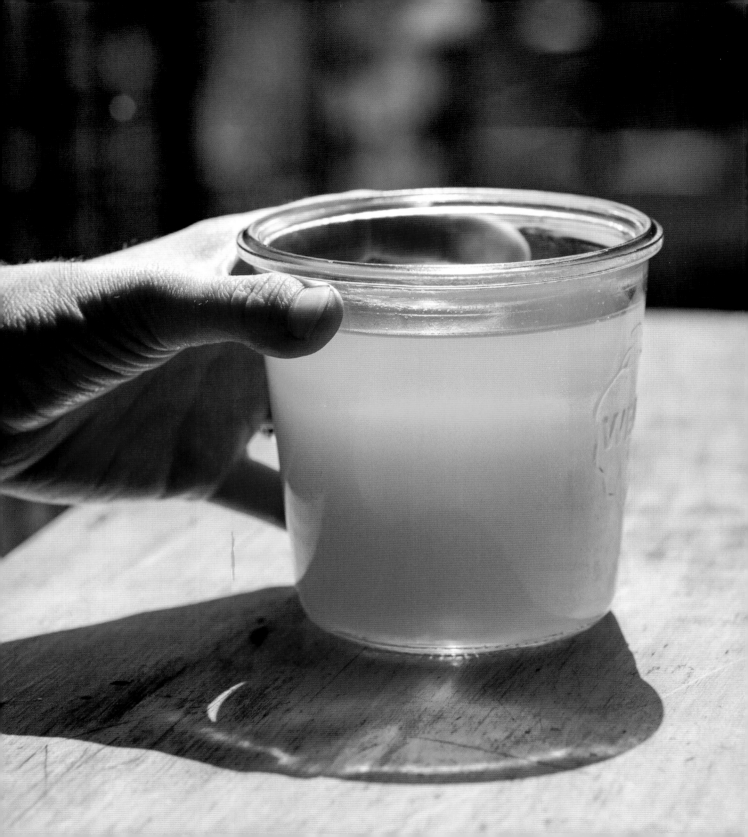

Homemade Bouillon:
Bone Broth to Go

WE LEARNED ABOUT THE ANCIENT TECHNIQUE TO make bouillon, before industrialization, from the blog of the wonderful and knowledgeable Jenny McGruther, called the Nourished Kitchen. Jenny explains that before the era of refrigeration, modern devices, and easy food access, travelers figured out how to make portable soup. They would simmer broth for hours, reducing it to produce a highly gelatinous broth. When cooled, it would turn into a firm and compact gel that could be cut into small pieces and dried for long-term storage. These pieces of gelled broth were easily portable and ready to eat with the addition of water.

The practical bouillon cubes that we know now are very poor renditions of the old versions. If you read the ingredients on the packaging of most conventional bouillon cubes, you will find that they are highly processed, with added MSG and hard-to-pronounce ingredients. These bouillon cubes also lack gelatin, the ingredient that gives broth one of its unique health-giving properties.

This recipe calls for a good-quality powdered gelatin to facilitate the texture necessary to make the broth portable. We have included a source in our Resource guide.

Bouillon

1 basic recipe beef, lamb, pork, chicken, turkey, or duck bone broth or 8 quarts broth

4 tablespoons powdered gelatin (use only if your basic broth recipe didn't yield a gelatinous broth)

1. Once you have cooked, cooled, and skimmed the broth, transfer it to a wide-mouth shallow pot. Simmer and reduce the broth to 2 cups. You will end up with a thick, syrupy broth. The time it takes to reduce the broth depends on the shape and depth of the pot. The wider and shallower it is, the less time it will take to reduce. Deep, narrow-mouth pots may take hours to reduce to 2 cups. We use 2 13-inch cast-iron pans to reduce 8 quarts of broth, and it takes about 3 ½ hours to reduce to 2 cups.

2. Turn off the heat and add the gelatin, if using, while the broth is still hot. Whisk vigorously and allow the broth to cool. Refrigerate overnight in a 8 × 8 inch square container.

3. At this point it will be easy to cut into 1 × 1 inch cubes. Each cube with added water makes a 1 cup serving of broth.

4. For longer storage, dry the bouillon cubes by wrapping in cloth and placing them in the refrigerator for at least 8 more hours. The cubes may be stored in the refrigerator up to 2 months or in the freezer for up to 1 year.

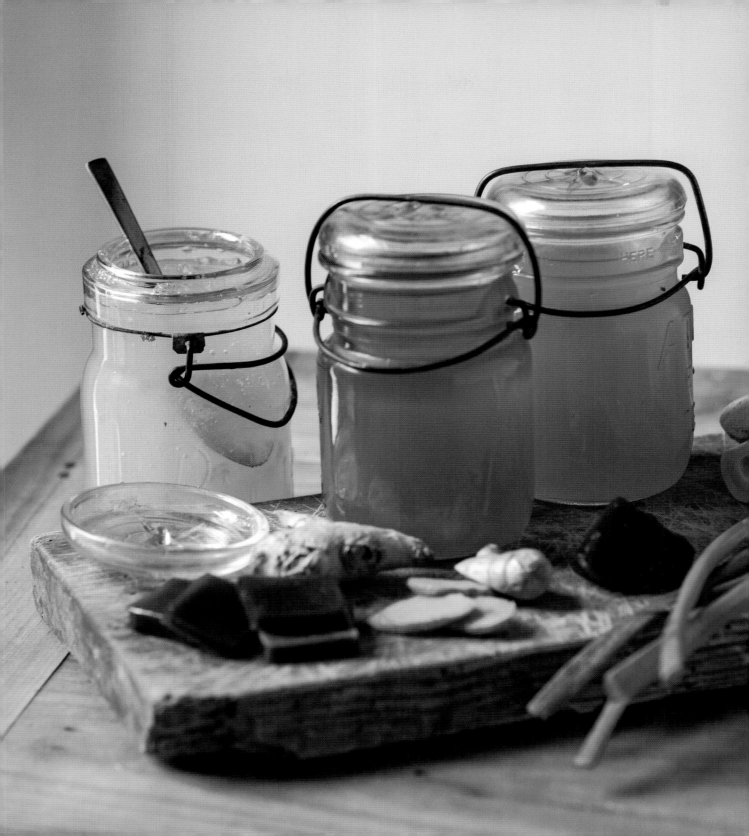

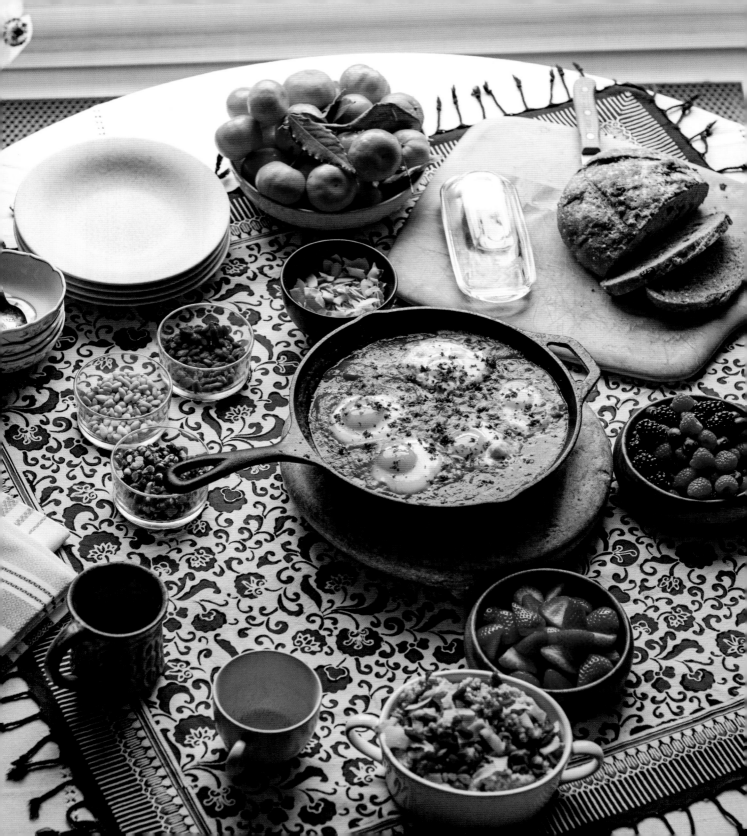

Resources

For herbs, spices, essential oils, seaweeds, culinary salts, and culinary oils:
https://www.mountainroseherbs.com

For carnaroli rice:
http://www.eataly.com

For wild-caught, sustainable fish:
http://www.vitalchoice.com

For wild prawns, clams, and squid:
http://www.marxfoods.com

For healthy fats and oils, salts and minerals, natural sweeteners, whole food supplements (including cod liver oil + high vitamin butter), water and air filtration systems, and nutrient-dense foods (including nuts, seeds, and butters):
http://www.radiantlifecatalog.com

For pasture-raised collagen and gelatin powders:
http://www.vitalproteins.com

For 12 ways to avoid toxins in the kitchen:
http://mightynest.com/learn/getting-started/healthy-living-guides/12-ways-to-avoid-toxins-in-the-kitchen

For 100 percent additive-free nutrients, formulas, and chemical-free body care:
http://www.drrons.com

To learn about the research of Weston Price and Francis Pottenger, and about food, lifestyle, healing modalities, and environmental practices for optimal health:
http://ppnf.org
http://www.westonaprice.org

For everything you need to know about pastured, unprocessed, full-fat milk:
http://www.realmilk.com

For research-based information about the benefits of choosing meat, eggs, and dairy products from pasture-raised animals:
http://www.eatwild.com

For recipes and information on nutrient-dense real and traditional foods:
http://nourishedkitchen.com

For organic chiles and organic beans:
http://www.marxfoods.com

For soap-making materials:
www.glorybee.com
www.enfleurage.com
www.mountainroseherbs.com

For coconut products:
http://www.tropicaltraditions.com

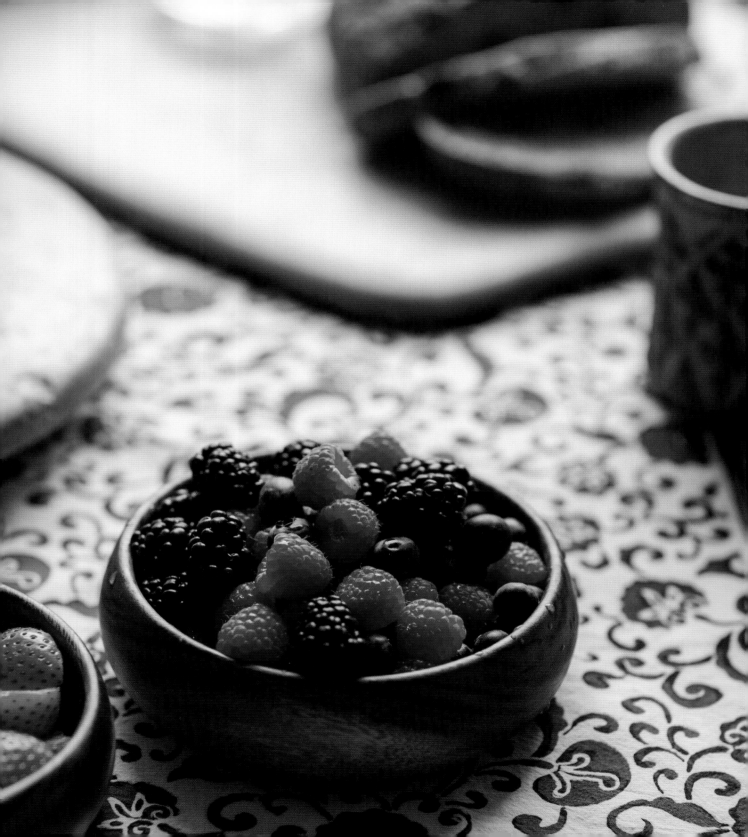

References and Suggested Reading

C. Agostini, B. Carratu, E. Riva, and E. Sanzini. "Free Amino Acid Content in Standard Infant Formulas: Comparison with Human Milk." *Journal of the American College of Nutrition* 19, no. 4 (2000): 434–438. doi:10.1080/07315724.2000.10718943. PMID 10963461.

Kaayla T. Daniel. "Bone Broth and MSG: What You Need to Know." The Healthy Home Economist website. http://www.thehealthyhomeeconomist.com/bone-broth-msg-what-you-need-to-know.

Sally Fallon and Mary G. Enig. "Feeding Babies." Weston A. Price Foundation website. December 31, 2001. http://www.westonaprice.org/health-topics/feeding-babies.

Sally Fallon and Mary G. Enig. *Nourishing Traditions: The Cookbook that Challenges Politically Correct Nutrition and the Diet Dictocrats.* White Plains, MD: NewTrends Publishing, 2001. 116–125.

Sally Fallon Morell and Kaayla T. Daniel. *Nourishing Broth: An Old-Fashioned Remedy for the Modern World.* New York: Hachette, 2014. 34–39.

Chris Kresser. "Ask the RD: Are Seeds Healthy and Animal Foods for Vegetarians." Chris Kresser website. February 17, 2014. http://chriskresser.com/ask-the-rd-are-seeds-healthy-and-animal-foods-for-vegetarians.

Chris Kresser. "Why Grass-Fed Trumps Grain-Fed." Chris Kresser website. March 29, 2013. http://chriskresser.com/why-grass-fed-trumps-grain-fed.

Jill C. Nienhiser. "About the Foundation." Weston A. Price Foundation website. January 1, 2000. http://www.westonaprice.org/about-the-foundation/about-the-foundation.

Will Revak and Susan Revak. "How Bone Broths Support Your Adrenals, Bones, and Teeth." Nourished Kitchen website. http://nourishedkitchen.com/bone-broths-adrenals-bones-teeth.

Katherine Zeratsky. "What Is MSG? Is It Bad for You?" Mayo Clinic website. http://www.mayoclinic.org/healthy-eating/expert-answers/monosodium-glutamate/gaq-20058196.

Yifang Zhang and Yingzhi Yao. *Your Guide to Health with Foods and Herbs: Using the Wisdom of Traditional Chinese Medicine.* New York: Better Link Press, 2012. 163–164.

Contributor

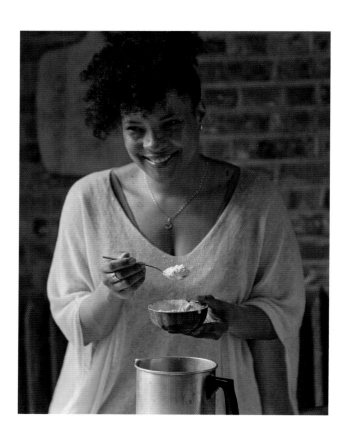

Erica Robinson

Erica Robinson is a soap expert and the owner of Amberkissed Soaps in New York City. She contributed the recipes for Tallow Soaps and Tallow Balms. Amberkissed is an Earth-sustainable company that focuses on apitherapy, aromatherapy, and the wonderful benefits of flowers, herbs, clays, natural oils, butters, and fats. Amberkissed joins Bone Deep & Harmony in the commitment to respect and use all available resources and reduce unnecessary waste.

Acknowledgments

WE'D LIKE TO EXTEND OUR GRATITUDE TO CHRIS Chen for introducing us to the healing power of bone broth. To both Chris and David Regellin, our partners, for still being our partners after we finally finished this! To Chris, David, Pablo, and Elsie as our resident, and always honest, taste testers. Teddy Mojica, Alberto Mojica, and Chad Davis for their photographs and vision. To Ted Smoot and Laura Frautschi and Cathy Zicherman for opening their beautiful homes to us to photograph this book. To Hilary Downes for holding our hand and sharing her savvy through the production of this project. To our parents and sisters for their unconditional support—Alberto Mojica, Christine Thompson, and Kristian Mojica-Vasudev, Kim, Jay, and Caroline Flynn. Geri Brewster for generously sharing her nutritional knowledge and supporting our business. Erica Robinson for her creative collaboration and friendship. To Marie Cudennec for her friendship, inspiration, and support across the pond. June Adams and the LEAAF daycare girls, for taking care of Pablo and Elsie and giving us the freedom to make this project happen. To Tim Forrester and the guys at Harlem Shambles for being game to experiment with us and giving us the opportunity to start Bone Deep & Harmony. To Jason Von Oijen for keeping us sane and in shape while we wrote this book. To Tamara Ljeskovac and Gabe Millman for gracefully manning the BD&H ship in our bookwriting absence. To Diana Ventimiglia and the dream team at Sterling behind this book for their trust in us and the opportunity to write this book.

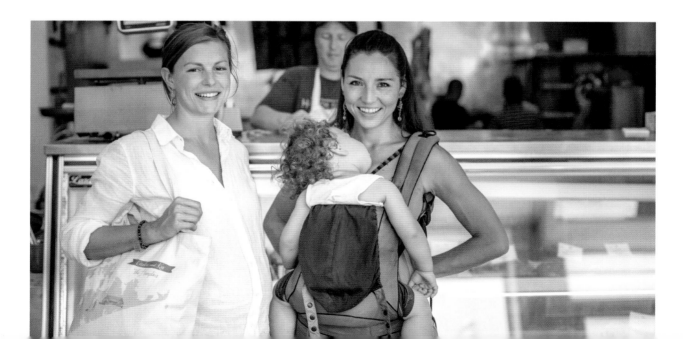

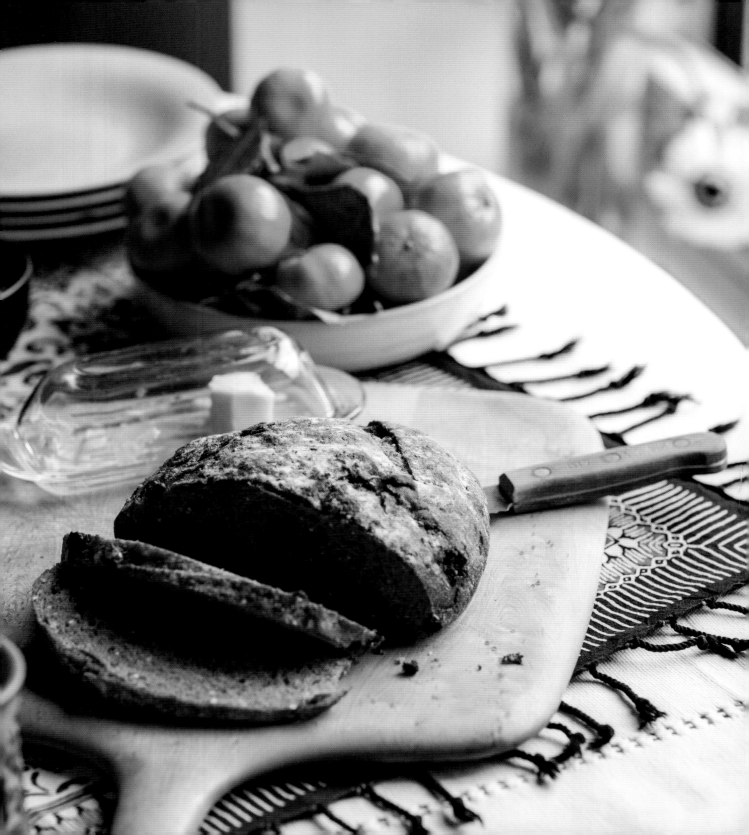

Praise

"The first time I drank broth was when I was 18 (I'm now 21) to alleviate some pretty persistent seasonal allergies and sneezing that I couldn't seem to shake. I drank one glass every morning, first thing, for about 10 days. The bone broth did the trick. The second round of "brothing" came this past year after an ugly episode of digestive confusion. For about 2 months I had to worry about vomiting every meal I ate an hour or so after eating it, no matter what it was. This all changed after going on a strict bone broth and chicken diet for 3 weeks . . . After going gung-ho with the bone broth, I had to slowly introduce different types of foods back into my diet. I started digesting those foods with great ease again. I felt better than I ever had before, without the slightest bit of nausea. A bonus of this improved digestion was the effect it had on my skin, my acne is now essentially non-existent."

—TIM BLAND, ACUPUNCTURE PATIENT AND
BONE DEEP & HARMONY CUSTOMER

"Bone Deep & Harmony's bone soup has done wonders for me, increasing my physical energy and sense of well-being, improved my pulse, made me more grateful to cows than I already was (how much we owe them!), and centered me in my daily practice."

—JANET, ACUPUNCTURE PATIENT AND
BONE DEEP & HARMONY CUSTOMER

"Bone Deep & Harmony's bone broth is like no other. Delicious and nourishing—my body actually craves it and my skin glows because of it! When I begin my day with bone broth, I have more energy and better digestion. It's magic. It's a great product sold by a superb company— caring and warm individuals who treat you right and are passionate about their product."

—NEENA B., BONE DEEP & HARMONY CUSTOMER

"In December of 2014, I was given a gift certificate by two fellow acupuncturists for the Bone Deep & Harmony Broth. As I was recovering from lymphoma, the impetus behind this generous holiday gift was to assist in rebuilding my health after intensive chemotherapy. As an acupuncturist, I recognize the importance of bone broth for it's nourishing and healing properties. Lya and Taylor were wonderful in their support and recommendations for a protocol for maximizing the benefits of the broth. After drinking 1 ½ cups daily for a 1 month, I started to notice a difference in the way I was feeling. Postchemotherapy I felt depleted, and both my stomach lining and tendons were compromised. The consistency of drinking the broth really helped me feel stronger and see improvements in my body. As per the girls' recommendation, I began to cook with the broth to better assimilate other foods. Currently I am in my third round of 12 quarts, and I have integrated the Bone Deep & Harmony Broth into my daily life. After my own positive experience, I have recommended the broth to my own patients. The health benefits are amazing and I am so thrilled that almost one year later, I am feeling great and am hooked on the broth! If you are considering trying the broth, take my advice . . . go for it . . . it's a game changer!"

—JAIME S. MARKS, LICENSED ACUPUNCTURIST AND
BONE DEEP & HARMONY CUSTOMER

"I choose Bone Deep & Harmony broth because I trust its conscientious production and lack of pretense; they are admittedly reviving an old tradition, and doing it in a way that is consistent with modern values about quality, environmental, and health concerns."

—HILARY DOWNES, BONE DEEP & HARMONY CUSTOMER

Index

Note: Page numbers in *italics* indicate photos on pages separate from recipes.

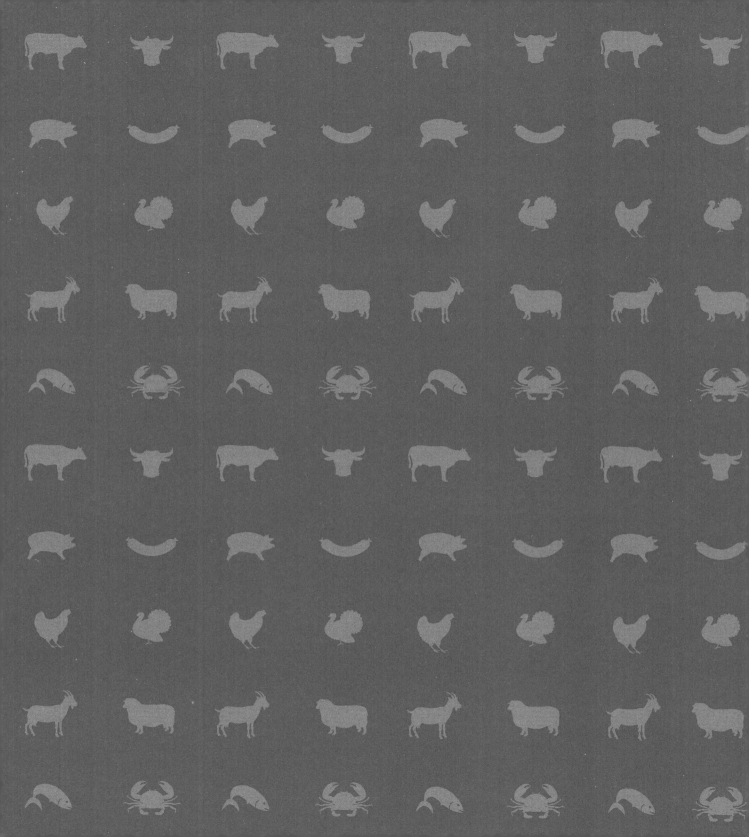